Neurotrauma

Samer S. Hoz · Iype Cherian · Ali A. Dolachee
Zahraa F. Al-Sharshahi · Hayder R. Salih
Mohammed A. Al-Rawi · Mohammed A. Al-Dhahir

Neurotrauma

In Multiple-Choice Questions

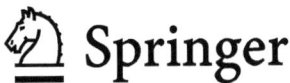 Springer

Samer S. Hoz
Department of Neurosurgery
Neurosurgery Teaching Hospital
Baghdad
Iraq

Ali A. Dolachee
Department of Surgery
University of Al-Qadisiyah
College of Medicine
Diwaniyah
Iraq

Hayder R. Salih
Department of Neurosurgery
Neurosurgery Teaching Hospital
Baghdad
Iraq

Mohammed A. Al-Dhahir
Department of Neurosurgery
Strong Memorial Hospital
Rochester, NY
USA

Iype Cherian
Department of Neurosciences
Krishna Institute of Medical Sciences
Malkapur
Maharashtra
India

Zahraa F. Al-Sharshahi
Department of Neurosurgery
Neurosurgery Teaching Hospital
Baghdad
Iraq

Mohammed A. Al-Rawi
Department of Neurosurgery
Neurosurgery Teaching Hospital
Baghdad
Iraq

ISBN 978-3-030-80868-6   ISBN 978-3-030-80869-3   (eBook)
https://doi.org/10.1007/978-3-030-80869-3

This Springer imprint is published by the registered company Springer Nature Switzerland AG
The registered company address is: Gewerbestrasse 11, 6330 Cham, Switzerland

To all neurosurgeons,
the unsung heroes who do more with less every day to continue serving our
people worldwide

To our patients,
who are our source of inspiration and the ultimate aim behind all our efforts

Foreword 1

About 5.48 million people are estimated to suffer from severe traumatic brain injury (TBI) each year (73 cases per 100,000 people). The WHO estimates that almost 90% of deaths due to injuries occur in low- and middle-income countries (LMICs), where the 85% of population live. Selection of patients is biased by the literature as 89% of published papers in TBI come from USA-Canada- Australia- Japan –Europe, where apparently is located less than 27 % of injuries. Moreover, there is evidence that even in high-income countries (HICs), there are conflicting guidelines at the regional/national and continental level because very few of the published guidelines have a solid evidence-based background. The only solution is to increase the grade of collaboration among HICs and LMICs to reach higher grade of evidence.

Thus, in the light of these considerations I want to express my gratitude to Dr. Hoz and his colleagues for considering me to give my opinion about this book. Maybe our respective workplaces could be different in terms of facilities; however the wish to share experiences, to give a high grade of neurosurgical training, is the same as anywhere. This book is testimony that limited material resources are less relevant when you have high cultural resources.

This manual could represent a stimulus to extend in deep the study of TBI and to encourage discussion with residents, young and expert neurosurgeons during the daily clinical practice and literature research. It doesn't replace classical neurosurgical manuals and books, but rather may act as an optimal educational tool for board exams due to the effective question and answer format, with succinct but detailed answers, covering the clinical aspects, diagnosis, and treatment.

The use of this book could be suggested even for neurologists and neuro-intensivists.

Corrado Iaccarino MD
Associate Professor,
Department of Biomedical, Metabolic and Neural Sciences,
University of Modena and Reggio Emilia,
Neurosurgery Division, University Hospital of Modena, Modena, Italy

Foreword 2

It is a pleasure to pen down a foreword note on this exciting book *Neurotrauma in Multiple Choice Questions* authored by Dr. Samer S. Hoz and his colleagues. Knowledge is acquired while searching and wisdom is acquired after experience. A brain twister is always challenging and interesting for a young student in neuroscience. Finding the correct answer need voracious reading and clear understanding of a subject. This is common for any subject, and when one finds the correct answer again and again, he or she can self-assess his or her knowledge in that particular subject. The multiple choice questions provide a great opportunity to rekindle the mind and search for the right answer. The authors have achieved their goal of providing an excellent manual for understanding neurotrauma through multiple choice questions in great detail. Neurotrauma is a vast subject and is commonly encountered by every neurosurgeon. The understanding of basics in neurotrauma is fast changing due to research, and the management protocols are seeing cascades of new developments in recent years. This manual with 3 sections, 8 chapters, and 400 MCQs is well crafted by the authors for the benefit of neurosurgery residents and young neurosurgeons all over the world. I wish the readers get benefited by this marvel by meticulously going through each question in detail. This manual not only provides an opportunity to learn more about neurotrauma but also will be a handy tool during examination and for self-assessment. My congratulations to all authors who worked hard to collect these pearls and the publishers for bringing in a great format.

Jutty K. B. C. Parthiban
Executive Member, Neurological Society India,
Asia Pacific Cervical Spine Society,
WFNS Spine Committee,
Head - Department of Neurosurgery,
Course Director - National Board Examination
for Neurosurgery, Kovai Medical Center Hospital,
Coimbatore, Tamil Nadu,
India

Foreword 3

I am delighted to write the foreword for the book *Neurotrauma in Multiple Choice Questions*. Dr. Samer S. Hoz is one of the most outstanding academic and clinic neurotrauma surgeons of our time. This book, based on multiple choice questions of neurotrauma, stands as a tribute to his dedication to excellence in traumatic neurosurgery. The book is based on the basic knowledge for making the management of the cranial neurotrauma, spinal neurotrauma, and peripheral neurotrauma. This book should be on the bookshelf of every neurosurgical trainee and practitioner and should be a required reading by everyone dealing with neurotrauma. The book contains a wealth of information in a concise, well-organized format.

Yonghong, Wang
Professor and Head, Neurotrauma Department, Shanxi Bethune Hospital, Shanxi Medical University Third Hospital, Taiyuan City, China

Preface

Dear reader,

We are delighted to introduce *Neurotrauma in Multiple Choice Questions* as your study companion.

The use of multiple-choice questions (MCQs) format for studying neurosurgery has the potential to solidify scientific information and identify knowledge gaps. It also allows for quick navigation through many topics in a timely manner, particularly when the questions are designed to include both common "must know" facts and the board-favorite challenging concepts.

Neurotrauma has been ingrained in the evolution of neurosurgery since its inception. Despite the evolution of distinct neurosurgical subspecialties, every practicing neurosurgeon must have a thorough understanding of the full spectrum of neurotrauma injuries.

The immediate beneficiaries of this work will be neurosurgery students, residents, fellows, and younger neurosurgeons preparing for board exams or practice.

The book should serve as a quick-access repository of board-favorite facts and practice essentials, assisting the reader in establishing a solid knowledge foundation and effortlessly retaining and recalling the information.

The book's sections take the reader through the fundamental principles of neurotrauma assessment, planning, decision-making, medical and surgical management, aftercare, and complication management. Each MCQs is designed to provide the reader with four correct facts and one false statement, as well as brief explanations to aid in consolidation.

We sincerely hope you enjoy and benefit from the book.

Samer S. Hoz
Baghdad, Iraq

Iype Cherian
Malkapur, Maharashtra, India

Ali A. Dolachee
Diwaniyah, Iraq

Zahraa F. Al-Sharshahi
Baghdad, Iraq

Hayder R. Salih
Baghdad, Iraq

Mohammed A. Al-Rawi
Baghdad, Iraq

Mohammed A. Al-Dhahir
Rochester, NY, USA

Key Features

— *Neurotrauma in Multiple Choice Questions* is the FIRST review book to use the multiple-choice question format in neurosurgical trauma. The aim of this book is to help readers revise the core concepts and maintain the knowledge of brain, spinal cord, and peripheral nerve trauma.

— The strategy and format of the questions provide a stepwise progression from definition to surgical decision-making, to provide a comprehensive and concise overview. This study companion is structured in three sections, with a total of eight chapters, including more than 350 MCQs in a convenient format that is suitable for self-study. Answers and explanations appear immediately below the questions to enhance readability.

— *Neurotrauma in Multiple Choice Questions* is written in accordance with the most up-to-date best practice evidence, with a style that mirrors the format adopted by the majority of local, regional, and international board examinations.

— The students of neurosurgery, the residents, the fellows, the younger neurosurgeons preparing for exams or practice, and even the later stage neurosurgeons are the target audience of this book.

— This subspecialty-focused MCQ book follows the concept and style of the internationally recognized book *Vascular Neurosurgery in Multiple Choice Questions*, authored by Dr. Samer S. Hoz (the first editor) and published by Springer.

— Each chapter also includes a collection of concise tables outlining the topic's pertinent classification, grading, and scoring systems.

— The reader is directed to a list of high-quality, peer-reviewed references at the end of each chapter corresponding to the topics covered in MCQs. In addition, at the end of the book, there is a "suggested reading book list" section that lists all highly recommended neurosurgery textbooks to provide a more detailed coverage of the topic addressed.

— This book is an adjunct to existing texts and does not intend to be the primary source of information; it rather aims to help readers identify their relevant strengths and weaknesses in the area.

— A focused end-of-chapter reference list is included to facilitate a more in-depth understanding of the topics covered. Finally, the book concludes with a list of high-priority neurosurgery textbooks for those interested in delving deeper into a particular area.

Contents

I   Cranial Neurotrauma

1   **Principles and Initial Assessment** 3
     Suggested Reading 23

2   **Management of Cranial Neurotrauma** 27
     Suggested Reading 46

3   **Complications, Outcome, and Other Aspects** 51
     Suggested Reading 61

II   Spinal Neurotrauma

4   **Principles and Initial Assessment** 65
     Suggested Reading 91

5   **Management of Spinal Neurotrauma** 95
     Suggested Reading 117

6   **Complications, Outcomes, and Other Aspects** 121
     Suggested Reading 129

III Peripheral Neurotrauma and Miscellaneous Issues

7   **Peripheral Nerve Neurotrauma** 133
     Suggested Reading 146

8   **Miscellaneous Issues Related to Neurotrauma** 149
     Suggested Reading 164

     Supplementary Information
     Suggested Reading Book List 168

Contributors

Abdullah H. Al Ramadan Pediatric Neurosurgery Department, Maternity and Children Hospital, First Health Cluster, Eastern Province, Saudi Arabia

Ahmed Nabil Department of Neurosurgery, St George's University Hospitals, NHS Foundation Trust, London, UK

Alaa H. Arkawazi Department of Neurosurgery, Neurosurgery Teaching Hospital, Baghdad, Iraq

Ali A. Dolachee Department of Surgery, University of Al-Qadisiyah, College of Medicine, Diwaniyah, Iraq

Ameya S. Kamat Macquarie University Hospital, Sydney, NSW, Australia

Awfa A. Aktham Department of Neurosurgery, Neurosurgery Teaching Hospital, Baghdad, Iraq

Baha'eddin A. Muhsen Rose Ella Burkhardt Brain Tumor and Neuro-Oncology Center, Neurological Institute, Cleveland Clinic, Cleveland, OH, USA

Bilal Ibrahim Braathen Neurological Center's Department of Neurosurgery, Cleveland Clinic, Weston, FL, USA

Elena Nestian Bagdasar Arseni Clinical Emergency Hospital, Bucharest, Romania

Eleni D-Tsianaka Department of Neurosurgery, Dar Al Shifa Hospital, Hawally, Kuwait

Fatima O. Ahmed College of Medicine, University of Al-Mustansiriyah, Baghdad, Iraq

Ghazwan Hazim Albu-Salih Department of Plastic and Reconstructive Surgery, Imam Ali General Hospital, Baghdad, Iraq

Haitham A. Obaid   Department of Neurosurgery, Neurosurgery Teaching Hospital, Baghdad, Iraq

Hayder R. Salih   Department of Neurosurgery, Neurosurgery Teaching Hospital, Baghdad, Iraq

Hazem Madi   Department of Neurosurgery, Jordan Hospital and Medical Centre, Amman, Jordan

Hira Burhan   Department of Neurosurgery, Institute of Neurosciences, Nobel Medical College and Teaching Hospital, Biratnagar, Nepal

Ignatius N. Esene   Neurosurgery Division, Faculty of Health Sciences, University of Bamenda, Bambili, Cameroon

Ismail Al-Kebsi   Yemeni German Hospital, Sana'a, Yemen

Iype Cherian   Department of Neurosciences, Krishna Institute of Medical Sciences, Malkapur, Maharashtra, India

Laith Thamir Al-Ameri   Department of Neurosurgery, Al-Kindy College of Medicine – University of Baghdad, Baghdad, Iraq

Margarida Silva Conceicao   Department of Neurosurgery, Centro Hospitalar Tondela e Viseu, Viseu Dão Lafões, Portugal

Maria Laura Laffitte   Department of Neurosurgery, Liverpool Hospital, Liverpool, UK

Mohammed A. Al-Dhahir   Department of Neurosurgery, Strong Memorial Hospital University of 15 Rochester, Rochester, NY, USA

Mohammed A. Al-Rawi   Department of Neurosurgery, Neurosurgery Teaching Hospital, Baghdad, Iraq

Mohammed A. Finjan   Department of ophthalmology, Ibn Al Haitham Teaching Eye Hospital, Baghdad, Iraq

Mohammed K. Alaskari Department of Trauma and Orthopedic Surgery, Al-Shaheed Ghazi Al-Hariri Hospital, Medical City, Baghdad, Iraq

Mohamed M. Arnaout Department of Neurosurgery, Zagazig University, Zagazig, Egypt

Mustafa M. Altaweel Department of Neurosurgery, Neurosurgery Teaching Hospital, Baghdad, Iraq

Mustafa Qusai Saoodi Department of Plastic and Reconstructive Surgery, Al-Wasity Teaching Hospital, Baghdad, Iraq

Mustapha Eyad College of Medicine, University of Baghdad, Baghdad, Iraq

Nawar Ghassan Department of Human Anatomy, Alrasheed University Medical College, Baghdad, Iraq

Rasha A. Alshakarchy Department of Neurosurgery, Neurosurgery Teaching Hospital, Baghdad, Iraq

Redab A. Alkhataybeh Department of Neurosurgery, Hashemite University, Zarqa, Jordan

Ruqayah A. Al-baidar College of Medicine, University of Baghdad, Baghdad, Iraq

Sama S. Albairmani College of Medicine, Universit of Al-Iraqia, Baghdad, Iraq

Samer S. Hoz Department of Neurosurgery, Neurosurgery Teaching Hospital, Baghdad, Iraq

Sarah A. Basindwah Department of Neurosurgery, King Khalid University Hospital at King Saud University, Riyadh, Saudi Arabia

Silky Chotai Department of Neurosurgery, Vanderbilt University Medical Center, Nashville, TN, USA

Taha Mohammed Algahoom Althawra Modern General Hospital, Sana'a, Yemen

Zahraa A. Alsubaihawi College of Medicine, University of Baghdad, Baghdad, Iraq

Zahraa F. Al-Sharshahi Department of Neurosurgery, Neurosurgery Teaching Hospital, Baghdad, Iraq

Zahraa M. Kareem College of Medicine, University of Baghdad, Baghdad, Iraq

Zaid S. Aljuboori Department of Neurosurgery, University of Washington, Seattle, WA, USA

Abbreviations

16MD-CTA	16-slice multidetector computed tomography angiography
ABC	Airway, breath, circulation
ABP	Arterial blood pressure
ACA	Anterior cerebral artery
ACDF	Anterior cervical discectomy and fusion
ACS	Anterior cord syndrome
ADH	Anti-diuretic hormone
ADI	Atlantodental interval
AKA	Also known as
ALL	Anterior longitudinal ligament
AOD	Atlanto-occipital dissociation
AOSPINE	Arbeitsgemeinschaft für Osteosynthesefragen—English translated to; working group for bone fusion issues
AP	Anterior posterior
Asdhs	Acute subdural hematoma
ASIA	American spinal injury association
ATCCS	Acute traumatic central cord syndrome
A-V	Arterio-venous
AVdO2	Arterial-jugular venous oxygen content difference
AVM	Arteriovenous malformation
BAI	Basion-axial interval
BCI	Blunt internal carotid artery injury
BCVI	Blunt cerebrovascular injury
BDI	Basion-dental interval
BMD	Bone marrow density
BP	Blood pressure
BS	Bulbocavernosus
BSCB	Blood-spinal cord barrier
BSS	Brown Sequard syndrome

C1 to C7	Cervical spine number
C8	Cervical nerve root number8
CBF	Cerebral blood flow
CCS	Central cord syndrome
CN	Cranial nerve
CNS	Central nervous system
CPP	Cerebral perfusion pressure
CRPS	Complex regional pain syndrome
CSDH	Chronic subdural hematoma
CSF	Cerebrospinal fluid
CSM	Cervical spondylotic myelopathy
C-spine	Cervical spine
CSW	Cerebral salt wasting
CSWS	Cerebral salt wasting syndrome
CT	Computerized tomography
CTA	CT angiography
CVP	Central venous pressure
CVS	Cardiovascular
DAI	Diffuse axial injury
DBS	Deep brain stimulation
DC	Decompressive craniectomy
DDR	Dead donor rule
DECRA	DECRA trial/2011 (Decompressive Craniectomy in Patients with Severe Traumatic Brain Injury)
DEXA	Dual energy X-ray absorptiometry
DI	Diabetes insipidus
DIC	Disseminated intravascular coagulation
DKA	Diabetic ketoacidosis
DSA	Digital subtraction angiography
DVT	Deep venous thrombosis
e.g.	For example
ECA	External carotid artery

EDH	Epidural hematoma
EDSs	Electro-diagnostic studies
EEG	Electroencephalography
EMG	Electromyography
EVD	External ventricular drain
FDA	Food and drug administration
fMRI	Functional magnetic resonance imaging
GCS	Glasgow Coma Scale
GFAP	Glial fibrillary acidic protein
GFB	Gunshot foreign body
GOS	Glasgow outcome score
GRE	Gradient echo
GSW	Gunshot wound
h	Hour
HF	Hangman fracture
HO	Heterotopic ossifications
HVM	High velocity missile
ICA	Internal carotid artery
ICH	Intracerebral hemorrhage
IC-HTN	Intracranial hypertension
ICP	Intracranial pressure
ICU	Intensive care unit
IL-6	Interleukin-6
ISP	Intraspinal pressure
IVC	Inferior vena cava
IVC	Intraventricular catheter
IVH	Intraventricular hemorrhage
K	Potassium
KE	Kinetic energy
L/P	Lactate/ pyruvate
L1 to L5	Lumber spine number
lb	Avoirdupois pound

LMWH	Low molecular weight heparin
LS	Lumber spine
MAP	Mean arterial pressure
MDD	Major depressive disorder
MLS	Midline shift
mm	Millimeters
mmhg	Millimeters of mercury
mosm/kg	Milliosmoles per kilogram
MRI	Magnetic resonance imaging
MRN	Magnetic resonance neurography
MVA	Motor vehicle accident
NASCIS	National Acute Spinal Cord Injury Study
NEXUS	National Emergency X-Ray Utilization Study
NG	Nasogastric
NICE	National Institute for health and Care Excellence
NPi	Neurological pupil index
NSAID	Non-steroidal anti-inflammatory drug
NSE	Neuron specific enolase
O.R.	Operation room
OCF	Occipital condyle fracture
PaCO2	Partial arterial pressure of carbon dioxide
PCWP	Pulmonary capillary wedge pressure
PE	Pulmonary embolism
PI	Povidone-iodine
PLC	The posterior ligament complex
PLL	Posterior longitudinal ligament
PMMA	Polymethylmethacrylate
PNS	Peripheral nervous system
PTS	Post-traumatic syringomyelia
RCT	Randomized control trials
RESCUEicp*	Randomized Evaluation of Surgery with Craniectomy for Uncontrollable elevation of intracranial pressure

S1 to S5	Sacral spine number
SAH	Subarachnoid hemorrhage
SCI	Spinal cord injury
SCIWORA	Spinal cord injury without radiographic abnormality
SCPP	Spinal cord perfusion pressure
SD	The standard deviation
SDH	Subdural hematoma
SED	Spinal epidural hematoma
SIADH	Syndrome of inappropriate anti-diuretic hormone
SLIC	Subaxial cervical spine injury classification
SPECT	Single photon emission computed tomography
SSRI	Selective serotonin receptor inhibitors
SSS	Superior sagittal sinus
STIR	Short tau inversion recovery
SVJO2	Jugular venous oxygen saturation
T1-T6	Thoracic vertebrae number one
T1W	T1 weighted image of MRI sequence
T2W	T2 weighted image of MRI sequence
TAL	Transverse atlantal ligament
TBI	Traumatic brain injury
TENS	Transcutaneous electrical nerve stimulation
TGF-B	Tumor growth factor-beta
TLICS	Thoracolumbar injury classification and severity score
TNF-a	Tumor necrotic factor-alpha
TON	Traumatic optic neuropathy
tSAH	Traumatic subarachnoid hemorrhage
UCH-L1	Ubiquitin C-terminal hydrolase L1
UTI	Urinary tract infection
V2	Segment 2 of vertebral artery
VA	Vertebral artery
VAI	Vertebral artery injury
VB	Vertebral body

WAD	Whiplash-associated disorder
WD	Wallerian degeneration
*RESCUEicp	(Trial of Decompressive Craniectomy for Traumatic Intracranial Hypertension).

Cranial Neurotrauma

Contents

Chapter 1   Principles and Initial Assessment – 3

Chapter 2   Management of Cranial
Neurotrauma – 27

Chapter 3   Complications, Outcome,
and Other Aspects – 51

Principles and Initial Assessment

Ahmed Nabil, Margarida Silva Conceicao,
Mohamed M. Arnaout, Zaid S. Aljuboori,
Zahraa F. Al-Sharshahi, Abdullah H. Al Ramadan,
Hayder R. Salih, and Iype Cherian

Contents

Suggested Reading – 23

© The Author(s), under exclusive license to Springer Nature Switzerland AG 2022
S. S. Hoz et al., *Neurotrauma*, https://doi.org/10.1007/978-3-030-80869-3_1

1

? 1. Posttraumatic cerebral edema.
The *FALSE* answer is:
A. Cytotoxic edema is due to injury of neurons or glia cells.
B. Cytotoxic edema occurs across a disrupted blood–brain barrier.
C. Vasogenic edema responds to corticosteroids.
D. A combination of cytotoxic and vasogenic edema is common.
E. The onset of edema is within hours of TBI.

✔ Answer B
- Cytotoxic edema occurs across an intact blood–brain barrier and is related to osmotic forces.

? 2. Malignant cerebral edema.
The *FALSE* answer is:
A. Could follow a gradual course from several days to a week
B. Increased cerebral blood volume
C. Loss of cerebrovascular autoregulation
D. Up to 100% mortality
E. More common in adults

✔ Answer E
- Malignant cerebral edema is more common in children.

? 3. Posttraumatic cytotoxic cerebral edema.
The *FALSE* answer is:
A. Water is driven across an intact blood–brain barrier
B. Common in brain tumors
C. Occurs at gray and white matter
D. Steroids are not effective
E. Diuretics are transiently effective

✔ Answer B
- Cytotoxic cerebral edema does not occur in tumors. Other etiologies include cerebral infarction, meningitis, diabetic ketoacidosis (DKA), and water intoxication.

? 4. Posttraumatic vasogenic cerebral edema.
The *FALSE* answer is:
A. Blood–brain barrier malfunction
B. Common in brain tumors
C. Occurs at white matter

D. Steroids are not effective
E. Diuretics are transiently effective

✅ **Answer D**
- Corticosteroids are effective in vasogenic cerebral edema. vasogenic cerebral edema is also frequently seen in brain tumors, abscesses, infarction, and TBI.

❓ **5. Cerebral herniation syndromes**
Cushing response. The *FALSE* answer is:
A. Associated with central herniation
B. Arterial hypotension
C. Bradycardia
D. Respiratory irregularity
E. Occurs in 33% of cases of intracranial hypertension

✅ **Answer B**
- Cushing's triad is arterial hypertension, bradycardia, and respiratory irregularity.

❓ **6. Cerebral herniation syndromes**
Central herniation. The *FALSE* answer is:
A. Downward shift of the brainstem toward the foramen magnum
B. Compresses perforating branches of basilar artery
C. Compromises the reticular formation in the midbrain and pons
D. Associated with Duret hemorrhage in the corpus callosum
E. May be associated with Parinaud syndrome

✅ **Answer D**
- Central (axial) herniation causes Duret hemorrhage in the brainstem.
- Duret hemorrhage is a small hemorrhage (or multiple hemorrhages) seen in the medulla or pons of patients with rapidly developping brain herniation rapidly developing brain herniation, especially central herniation. Durent hemorrhage is most commonly seen in patients with severe herniation 12–24 hours prior to death.
- Parinaud syndrome, also known as the dorsal midbrain syndrome, is a supranuclear vertical gaze disturbance caused by compression of the superior tectal plate. Parinaud syndrome is characterized by a classic triad of findings: upward gaze palsy, pupillary light-near dissociation, and convergence-retraction nystagmus.

1

⑦ 7. Cerebral herniation syndromes

Subfalcine herniation. The *FALSE* answer is:

A. Herniation of the cingulate gyrus under the falx cerebri
B. The most common herniation syndrome
C. May result in upper limb monoparesis
D. May result in paraparesis
E. Compresses pericallosal arteries

✅ Answer C

━ Lower limb monoparesis. The lower extremity is the most commonly associated with anterior cerebral artery (ACA) syndrome or sometimes the deficit is hemiparesis of lower more than upper limb.

⑦ 8. Cerebral herniation syndromes

Uncal (trans-tentorial) herniation. The *FALSE* answer is:

A. Uncal and hippocampal herniation into the ambient and crural cisterns
B. Caused by mass lesions in the lateral middle fossa
C. Causes contralateral hemiparesis
D. Causes contralateral oculomotor nerve palsy
E. May cause Kernohan's notch phenomena

✅ Answer D

━ Uncal herniation causes ipsilateral oculomotor nerve palsy, contralateral paresis, and coma.

━ Kernohan's notch phenomenon is an imaging finding resulting from extensive midline shift due a mass effect, resulting in the indentation in the contralateral cerebral crus by the tentorium cerebelli. Causes hemiparesis that is ipsilateral to the expanding mass which is a false localizing sign.

⑦ 9. Cerebral herniation syndromes

Tonsillar herniation. The *FALSE* answer is:

A. Prolapse of the cerebellar tonsils through the foramen magnum
B. Compresses the midbrain
C. Causes hypertension
D. Causes bradypnea
E. Causes cardiorespiratory arrest and death

✅ Answer B

━ Tonsillar herniation compresses the medulla oblongata and, in some cases, the upper cervical cord.

? **10. Cerebral herniation syndromes**
   Ascending trans-tentorial herniation. The *FALSE* answer is:
   A. Also known as reverse herniation
   B. Cerebellar tonsils ascend through the tentorial hiatus
   C. Compress the midbrain
   D. Compress superior cerebellar arteries
   E. Occurs in posterior fossa masses and exacerbated by ventriculostomy

✅ **Answer B**
   – Ascending tenstentorial herniation is the herniation of cerebellar vermis upward through tentorial hiatus.

? **11. Neurological examination in TBI**
   Pupils. The *FALSE* answer is:
   A. Pons lesion: bilateral pinpoint pupils
   B. Midbrain lesion: bilateral fixed and dilated pupils
   C. Medulla lesion: bilateral fixed and dilated pupils
   D. Occipital lobe lesion: Bilateral fixed and dilated pupil
   E. Brain death: bilateral fixed and dilated pupils

✅ **Answer D**
   – Occipital lobe lesions result in unilateral fixed dilated pupil.

? **12. Neurological examination in TBI**
   Horner syndrome. The *FALSE* answer is:
   A. Involves the sympathetic pathway
   B. Indicates carotid dissection
   C. Represents a postganglionic injury
   D. Anhidrosis may be absent
   E. The miotic pupil is the normal one

✅ **Answer E**
   – In Horner syndrome, the miotic (smaller) pupil is the abnormal one. Posttraumatic Horner syndrome represents a third-order neuron disorder with injury to the postganglionic neurons at the level of the internal carotid artery. Anhidrosis is usually limited or absent. The Paredrine test helps to localize the cause of the miosis. If the third-order neuron is intact, then the amphetamine causes neurotransmitter

1

vesicle release, thus releasing norepinephrine into the synaptic cleft and resulting in robust mydriasis of the affected pupil. If the lesion itself is of the third-order neuron, then the amphetamine will have no effect and the pupil will remain constricted.

❷ 13. Neurological examination in TBI
Gaze deviation. The *FALSE* answer is:
A. Irritative frontal lesion: deviation away from the lesion
B. Irritative pontine lesion: deviation away from lesion
C. Midbrain pretectal lesion: upward gaze palsy
D. Medial thalamic hemorrhage: the "wrong way gaze"
E. Oculomotor nerve palsy: deviation down and out

✔ Answer B
— An irritative pontine lesion will result in eye deviation toward the side of the lesion.
— In supratentorial (frontal lobe) lesions, the deviation is towards the side of a destructive lesion and away from that of an irritative lesion.
— In infratentorial (pontine) lesions, the deviation is toward irritative lesions and away from destructive lesions.
— In median thalamic hemorrhage, the eyes will deviate away from the side of the lesion (wrong gaze palsy).
— Abducens nerve plasy will cause the ipsilateral eye to deviate inwards.
— Midbrain (pre-tectal lesions) are associated with an upward gaze plasy (Parinaud's syndrome).

❷ 14. Neurological examination in TBI
Parinaud's syndrome etiologies. The *FALSE* answer is:
A. Thalamic lesion
B. Midbrain pretectal lesion
C. Barbiturates coma
D. Seizures
E. Tumors of pons

✔ Answer E
— Pineal tumors NOT pons.

❓ 15. Answer A: Respiratory patterns in coma.
The *FALSE* answer is:
 A. Bilateral hemispheric: Cheyne-Stokes
 B. Thalamus: Kussmaul
 C. Midbrain: Hyperventilation
 D. Pons: Apneustic
 E. Medullary: Ataxic

✅ Answer B
 ▬ Kussmaul's breathing is nonspecific and occurs in severe acidosis, as in alcohol ingestion, uremia, and DKA.

❓ 16. Neurological examination in coma
The *FALSE* answer is:
 A. Arms extend and legs flaccid in decorticate posturing
 B. Decorticate posturing occurs in large cortical lesions
 C. Decerebrate posturing occurs in lesions below the lower midbrain
 D. Arms flexed and legs flaccid in pontine tegmentum lesions
 E. Decerebrate has a worse prognosis than decorticate posturing

✅ Answer A
 ▬ Arms flex and legs extend in decorticate posturing.

❓ 17. Brain death
The *FALSE* answer is:
 A. Absent gag reflex
 B. Dilated fixed pupils
 C. Positive occulocephalic reflex
 D. Absent corneal reflex
 E. Absent cough reflex

✅ Answer C
 ▬ Negative (absence) occulocephalic reflex is a sign of brainstem death.

❓ 18. Caloric testing (oculovestibular reflex)
The *FALSE* answer is:
 A. Records the function of each labyrinth separately
 B. Can be done with water or air
 C. Differentiates central from peripheral lesions
 D. Normal test: eyes deviate toward the cold stimulus
 E. Abnormal test: eyes deviate away from the warm stimulus

1

✅ **Answer D**

— Remember COWS (Cold-Opposite, Warm-Same) which represents normal testing. The caloric test will be abnormal in brain death, that is, Cold-Same, Warm-Opposite. The test can be made with ice or warm water which is irrigated inside the external auditory canal. In the absence of tympanic lesions, with the head of bed elevated to 30 degrees.

❓ **19. The oculocephalic reflex**
  The *FALSE* answer is:
  A. An application of the vestibular-ocular reflex
  B. Contraindicated in suspected C-spine injury
  C. Eyes rotate opposite to head direction: abnormal brainstem function
  D. Eyes rotate opposite to head direction: normal brainstem function
  E. A similar examination is performable for vertical eye movements

✅ **Answer C**

— In brain death, there will be loss of brainstem function, meaning that the eyes will move to the same side of head movement.

❓ **20. Indications for head CT scan within the first hour following TBI.**
  The *FALSE* answer is:
  A. GCS < 13 on initial assessment
  B. Posttraumatic seizure
  C. Suspected depressed skull fracture
  D. Head injury in patients on warfarin
  E. Large scalp laceration

✅ **Answer E**

❓ **21. Indications for head CT scan within 8 hours of TBI**
  The *FALSE* answer is:
  A. Loss of consciousness
  B. Above 65 years
  C. History of bleeding disorder
  D. Dangerous mechanism of injury
  E. Less than 30 min of retrograde amnesia

✅ **Answer E**

— No criteria for a head CT scan after a brief retrograde amnesia in isolation.

❓ 22. TBI. Rotterdam CT score

The *FALSE* answer is:

A. Depressed skull fracture
B. Midline shift
C. Epidural mass lesion
D. Intraventricular hemorrhage
E. Subarachnoid hemorrhage

✅ Answer A

– Skull fractures are not included in the Rotterdam classification.

❓ 23. TBI. Rotterdam CT score

The *FALSE* answer is:

A. Absent cisterns: 2 points
B. Normal cisterns: 0 points
C. Compressed cisterns: 1 point
D. Intraventricular hemorrhage present: 1 point
E. Epidural mass lesion present: 1 point

✅ Answer E

– The presence of epidural mass equals zero points, while their absence gives 1 point.
– Rotterdam score is aimed at improving prognostic evaluation of patients admitted with acute traumatic brain injuries.

Rotterdam score.

Predictor value	Score
Basal cistern	
Normal	0
Compressed	1
Absent	2
Midline shift	
No or <5 mm	0
Shift >5 mm	1
Epidural mass lesion	
Present	0
Absent	1

1

Predictor value	Score
Intraventricular blood or tSAH	
Absent	0
Present	1
Sum score	+1
tSAH: Traumatic subarachnoid hemorrhage	

? 24. TBI. Marshall CT classification
The *FALSE* answer is:
A. Marshal I: No lesion
B. Marshal II: Diffuse injury
C. Marshal III: Diffuse injury with swelling
D. Marshal IV: Diffuse injury with shift
E. Marshal VI: Evacuated mass lesion

✔ Answer E
- Marshal V: Evacuated mass lesion. Marshal VI: Nonevacuated mass lesion.
- Marshal classification serves as an outcome prediction tool in TBI patients.

Marshall classification

Classification	Description	Mortality
I	No lesion in CT	6.4%
II - diffuse injury	MLS 0–5 mm Visible basal cisterns No high or mixed density lesions ≥ 25 cm[a]	11%
III - diffuse injury swelling	MLS 0–5 mm Compressed/effaced basal cisterns No high or mixed density lesions ≥ 25 cm[a]	29%
IV - diffuse injury Shift	MLS >5 mm No high or mixed density lesions ≥ 25 cm[a]	44%
V - Evacuated mass lesion	Any lesion evacuated surgically	30%
VI - nonevacuated mass lesion	High or mixed density lesions ≥ 25 cm Not surgically evacuated lesion	34%

[a]Estimated volume, may include bone fragments and foreign bodies

❓ 25. TBI. Multimodality monitoring
The *FALSE* answer is:
A. Central venous pressure
B. Jugular bulb venous oximetry
C. Intracranial pressure
D. Lactate/glucose ratio
E. Brain tissue oxygen tension

✅ Answer A
- Central venous pressure is NOT a method of multimodality monitoring in TBI.
- Multimodality neuromonitoring in traumatic brain injury (TBI) includes glycerol, glucose, lactate/pyruvate ratio, lactate/glucose ratio, glutamate, near-infrared spectroscopy, Jugular bulb venous oximetry, intracranial pressure (ICP) monitoring, brain tissue oxygen tension, cerebral perfusion pressure (CPP), pressure reactivity index, and other noninvasive ICP monitoring methods.

❓ 26. TBI. Multimodality neuromonitoring
The *FALSE* answer is:
A. Pressure reactivity index: correlation between arterial blood pressure (ABP) and ICP
B. Cerebral ischemia in severe TBI decreases the lactate/pyruvate (L/P) ratio
C. Jugular bulb venous oximetry: global cerebral oxygenation and metabolism
D. Brain tissue oxygen tension: availability of oxygen for oxidative energy metabolism
E. CPP is calculated by subtracting mean ICP from mean ABP.

✅ Answer B
- Cerebral ischemia and increased anaerobic respiration increase the L/P ratio and relate to poor neurologic outcomes.

❓ 27. TBI. Cerebral microdialysis
The *FALSE* answer is:
A. Found after cell injury
B. Systemic lipolysis may affect its cerebral levels
C. Released from phospholipids following cell membrane degradation
D. Low extracellular glucose levels are associated with good outcome
E. Reduced CBF (ischemia) may decrease its extracellular concentration

✅ **Answer D**

- Reduced cerebral blood flow (CBF) (ischemia) or increased consumption of glucose may lead to a decrease in glycerol extracellular concentration. Low extracellular glucose levels are associated with poor outcome after TBI.

❓ **28. Jugular venous oxygen saturation SVJO2**

The *FALSE* answer is:

A. SjVO2 ≥ 55–75%: normal
B. SjVO2 < 50%: ischemia
C. Multiple desaturations: poor outcome
D. Sustained desaturations: evaluate for correctable causes
E. High SjVO2 > 75%: good outcome

✅ **Answer E**

- High SjVO2 > 75% may indicate hyperemia or infarcted tissue and is associated with poor outcomes. Other causes of desaturation include increased ICP, poor catheter position, CPP < 60 mmHg, surgical lesions, and $PaCO_2$ < 28 mmHg

❓ **29. Arterial-jugular venous oxygen content difference (AVdO2).**

The *FALSE* answer is:

A. AVdO2 of 6.5 vol %: normal
B. AVdO2 > 9 ml/dl: global cerebral ischemia
C. AVdO2 > 4 ml/dl: cerebral hyperemia
D. AVdO2 is independent of CBF
E. AVdO2 < 4 ml/dl: luxury reperfusion

✅ **Answer C**

- AVdO2 < 4 ml/dl indicates cerebral hyperemia.

❓ **30. ICP measurement**

The *FALSE* answer is:

A. Mean arterial pressure (MAP) = diastolic pressure + 1/3 pulse pressure
B. Normal adult ICP: 7–15 mmHg
C. Normal adult CPP is >50 mmHg
D. Standing adult ICP of −10 is normal
E. CPP has to drop below 70 before CBF would be impaired

✅ **Answer E**

- Due to cerebral autoregulation, CPP has to drop below 40 before CBF if affected.

❓ 31. ICP monitoring: indications
  The *FALSE* answer is:
  A. Severe TBI: GCS ≤ 8
  B. Normal brain computerized tomography (CT) with drowsiness only
  C. Multiple systems injury with altered consciousness
  D. Post hematoma evacuation
  E. Abnormal brain CT with cerebral edema

✅ Answer B
  ▬ Normal brain CT with ≥2 of the risk factors for intracranial hypertension (IC-HTN) is an indication of ICP monitoring. Add risk factors.
  ▬ Up to 50% of patients who subsequently develop increased ICP may have a normal admission head CT scan. In these patients, an ICP monitor is recommended if two or more of the following are present at admission: age >40 years, unilateral or bilateral motor posturing, or episodes of systolic blood pressure <90 millimeters of mercury (mmHg).

❓ 32. ICP monitoring devices
  The *FALSE* answer is:
  A. Intraparenchymal monitor is the most accurate.
  B. EVD allows CSF drainage.
  C. EVD must be maintained at a fixed reference point.
  D. In subarachnoid bolt, high ICP causes false low readings.
  E. Open anterior fontanelle can be used in infants.

✅ Answer A
  ▬ Intraventricular catheter (IVC): also known as (AKA) external ventricular drain (EVD) is the most accurate device for ICP monitoring.

❓ 33. ICP monitoring devices: Intraventricular catheter (IVC)
  The *FALSE* answer is:
  A. Can be used in children
  B. Utilizes transducers tipped with fiber optic devices
  C. Is the most accurate
  D. Can not be recalibrated
  E. Allows CSF drainage

✅ Answer D
  ▬ IVC has the lowest cost. It is the most accurate and can be recalibrated to minimize measurement drift.

1

? 34. Secondary Intracranial Hypertension: Causes
  The *FALSE* answer is:
  A. Hyperventilation
  B. Delayed hematoma formation
  C. Cerebral vasospasm
  D. Delayed edema formation
  E. Hyponatremia

✓ Answer A
  ▬ Hyperventilation is not a cause of secondary IC-HTN. Hypoventilation can be a cause of secondary IC-HTN. A secondary increase in ICP is sometimes observed 3–10 days following the trauma.

? 35. ICP waveforms
  The *FALSE* answer is:
  A. Can be used to predict raised ICP
  B. Respiratory variations affect normal waveforms
  C. Plateau waves: ICP elevations ≥30 mmHg for 5–20 minutes
  D. Abnormal B wave lasts for 30 seconds–2 minutes
  E. Low-amplitude C waves are sometimes normal

✓ Answer C
  ▬ Plateau waves occur when ICP is ≥50 mmHg for 5–20 minutes.

? 36. ICP waveforms
  The *FALSE* answer is:
  A. Type A wave is synonymous with Traube–Hering waves.
  B. Normal ICP waveforms are small pulsations transmitted from the systemic blood pressure into the intracranial cavity.
  C. The large (1–2 mmHg) peak corresponds to the arterial systolic pressure wave, with a small dicrotic notch.
  D. The central venous "A" wave is from the right atrium.
  E. Expiration causes ICP elevation.

✓ Answer A
  ▬ Type C wave is also known as Traube–Hering waves.

? 37. ICP waveforms
  The *FALSE* answer is:
  A. As ICP rises and cerebral compliance decreases, the arterial pulses become more pronounced.

B. In right atrial cardiac insufficiency, the CVP rises and the ICP waveform takes on a more "venous" appearance.
C. In right atrial cardiac insufficiency, the venous "A" wave begins to predominate.
D. Plateau waves are usually aborted at the onset by instituting treatments.
E. The Lundberg D wave is associated with higher morbidity rates.

✅ **Answer E**

Types of Lundberg waves:
- **Lundberg A waves** AKA plateau waves of Lundberg: ICP elevations ≥50 mmHg for 5–20 minutes. Usually accompanied by a simultaneous increase in MAP (it is debated whether the latter is cause or effect)
- **Lundberg B waves** AKA pressure pulses: amplitude of 10–20 mmHg is lower than A waves. Variation with types of periodic breathing. Lasts 30 seconds–2 minutes.
- **Lundberg C waves**: frequency of 4–8/minute. Low-amplitude C waves (AKA Traube–Hering waves) may sometimes be seen in the normal ICP waveform. High-amplitude C waves may be pre-terminal and may sometimes be seen on top of plateau waves.

❓ **38. TBI. Syndrome of inappropriate anti-diuretic hormone (SIADH)**
The *FALSE* answer is:
A. Hyponatremia
B. Hypovolemia
C. Serum osmolality <275 milliosmoles per kilogram (mOsm/kg)
D. High urinary osmolality
E. Normal renal function

✅ **Answer B**
- Syndrome of inappropriate anti-diuretic hormone (SIADH) is characterized by euvolemia (or hypervolemia). SIADH is caused by the release of anti-diuretic hormone (ADH) in the absence of physiologic (osmotic) stimuli. Diagnostic criteria include hyponatremia, inappropriately concentrated urine, and no evidence of renal or adrenal dysfunction.

❓ **39. TBI. Cerebral salt wasting syndrome (CSWS)**
The *FALSE* answer is:
A. Hyponatremia
B. Hypovolemia
C. High/normal serum K

D. High serum osmolality
E. Dehydration

✅ **Answer D**
- In CSW, the serum osmolarity is low.

❓ **40. TBI. CSWS**
   The *FALSE* answer is:
   A. Low central venous pressure (CVP)
   B. Decreased serum potassium
   C. Hyponatremia
   D. Low pulmonary capillary wedge pressure (PCWP)
   E. Low plasma volume

✅ **Answer B**
- CSWS is associated with normal-high serum potassium levels.

❓ **41. CSW versus SIADH**
   The *FALSE* answer is:
   A. The plasma volume is higher in CSWS.
   B. The salt balance is normal in SIADH.
   C. PCWP is low in CSWS.
   D. CVP is low in CSWS.
   E. Orthostatic hypotension occurs in both.

✅ **Answer A**
- The plasma volume is lower in CSWS.
- To compare between CSW and SIADH, the two most important differences are extracellular volume and salt balance. An elevated serum [K+] with hyponatremia is incompatible with the diagnosis of SIADH.

❓ **42. CSW versus SIADH**
   The *FALSE* answer is:
   A. High hematocrit in CSWS
   B. Lower urinary salt CSWS
   C. Serum potassium (K) is elevated in CSWS
   D. Normal serum uric acid in CSWS
   E. Normal serum uric acid in SIADH

✔ **Answer B**
- Urinary salt is two times higher in CSWS.

❓ **43. TBI. Diabetes insipidus**
The *FALSE* answer is:
A. Low ADH levels
B. Craving for water
C. High output of dilute urine
D. Normal or high serum Na
E. Adrenal insufficiency

✔ **Answer E**
- Normal adrenal function in DI as it cannot occur in primary adrenal insufficiency because a minimum of mineralocorticoid activity is needed for the kidney to make free water.

❓ **44. TBI. Diabetes insipidus (DI)**
The *FALSE* answer is:
A. Central DI: subnormal levels of ADH
B. Inability to concentrate urine to >300 mOsm/kg
C. Large doses of mannitol can mimic it
D. Low serum sodium
E. Normal adrenal function

✔ **Answer D**
- Central DI is characterized by normal or above-normal serum sodium.

❓ **45. Pediatric TBI**
The *FALSE* answer is:
A. Central nervous system (CNS) injuries are the most common cause of traumatic death
B. Subgaleal hematoma is usually soft, fluctuant
C. Subperiosteal hematoma extend over skull sutures
D. Growing skull fractures require a widely separated fracture and a dural tear
E. A ping pong fracture is seen only in the newborn

1

✅ **Answer C**
- Subperiosteal hematoma is limited by skull sutures.

❓ **46. Subgaleal hematoma in children**
The *FALSE* answer is:
A. Bleeding between the galea from periosteum
B. Limited by suture lines
C. Usually starts as a small localized hematoma
D. Under one year of age significant loss of circulating blood volume
E. Soft fluctuant mass

✅ **Answer B**
- Subgaleal hematoma may cross sutures.

❓ **47. Subperiosteal hematoma in children**
The *FALSE* answer is:
A. Commonly seen in newborns
B. Limited by sutures
C. Firmer than subgaleal hematoma
D. Scalp moves freely over the mass
E. Does not reabsorb

✅ **Answer E**
- 80% reabsorb, usually within 2–3 weeks. Occasionally may calcify.

❓ **48. Growing skull fractures (posttraumatic leptomeningeal cysts)**
The *FALSE* answer is:
A. Nondisplaced, linear skull fracture is typical
B. Requires a dural tear
C. Over 90% occur before 3 years
D. Parietal is the most common location
E. Surgery must involve dural repair

✅ **Answer A**
- Growing skull fractures are characterized by bone diastasis 3 mm or more.
- The most common age group is 3 months to 3 years.

49. Nonaccidental head injury in pediatrics
   The *FALSE* answer is:
   A. Retinal hemorrhage
   B. Ping pong fracture
   C. Multiple injuries of different ages
   D. Bilateral CSDH in a child <2 years of age
   E. Significant neurological injury with minimal external trauma

Answer B
 — The "ping pong fracture" is not a factor of suspected child abuse. Unlike in accidental TBI in children, skull fractures are not typically located at the frontal bone in nonaccidental trauma.
 — "Ping pong ball" fracture: A green-stick type of fracture → caving in of a focal area of the skull as in a crushed area of a ping pong ball. Usually is seen only in the newborn due to the plasticity of the skull. Retinal hemorrhages, subdural hematomas (bilateral in 80%), and/or subarachnoid hemorrhage (SAH) are frequently found in these cases.

50. Pediatric retinal hemorrhage
   The *FALSE* answer is:
   A. Clears slower than preretinal hemorrhage
   B. Inflicted versus accidental injury can be differentiated
   C. Causes: acute high-altitude sickness
   D. Causes: acute increase in ICP
   E. Frequently associated with intracerebral hemorrhage (ICH)

Answer A
 — Retinal hemorrhage clears much faster than preretinal hemorrhage.
 — In a traumatized child with multiple injuries and an inconsistent history, the presence of retinal hemorrhage is pathognomonic for child abuse.

51. Penetrating TBI
   The *FALSE* answer is:
   A. Less prevalent than closed TBI
   B. Mostly caused by low-velocity objects
   C. Mechanisms include cavitation and shockwaves
   D. Brain damage depends on the kinetic energy imparted
   E. Velocity has greater influence than projectile mass

1

✅ **Answer B**

 — In the civilian population, TBI is mostly caused by high-velocity objects.

❓ **52. Penetrating TBI. Factors associated with higher mortality**

The *FALSE* answer is:
A. Traverses the ventricles
B. High-velocity projectiles
C. Crosses the midline
D. Tangential injuries
E. Large missiles

✅ **Answer D**

 — Tangential injuries are associated with lower mortality rates.

❓ **53. Blunt Cerebrovascular injury (BCVI): risk factors**

The *FALSE* answer is:
A. Basilar skull fracture involving the carotid canal
B. GCS < 6.
C. CSF rhinorrhea
D. Cervical vertebral body fracture
E. Fractures involving C1–3

✅ **Answer C**

 — CSF rhinorrhea is a sign of skull base fracture and is not a risk factor for BCVI.
 — Cervical fractures at any level, but specially C1 to C3 + transverse foramen fracture, subluxation, or ligamentous injury at any level and/or near hanging lesion with are all risk factors for BCVI

❓ **54. BCVI: signs and symptoms**

The *FALSE* answer is:
A. Nasal arterial hemorrhage
B. Cervical bruit in a patient <50 years old
C. Expanding cervical hematoma
D. Focal neurological deficits
E. Neurological deficit with head CT abnormalities

✅ **Answer E**

 — Neurologic deficit **without** head CT alterations.

❓ 55. BCVI: Denver grading scale

The *FALSE* answer is:
- A. Luminal irregularity with <25% stenosis is Grade I.
- B. ≥25% luminal stenosis is Grade II.
- C. 16-slice multidetector CT angiography is equivalent to catheter angiography in BCVI diagnosis.
- D. The Denver grade of the dissection correlates the risk of stroke from ICA dissection.
- E. Intraluminal thrombus alone is Grade V.

✔ Answer E
- ▬ Intraluminal thrombus is Grade II, while transection with free extravasation is Grade V.

\ BCVI grading scale ("Denver grading scale")	
Grade	**Description**
I	luminal irregularity with <25% stenosis
II	≥25% luminal stenosis or intraluminal thrombus or raised intimal flap
III	pseudoaneurysm
IV	occlusion
V	transection with free extravasation

- ▪ **Imaging recommendations for BVI Detection:**
  1. 16MD-CTA should be obtained as follows:
     - ▬ Emergently in patients with signs/symptoms of BCVI
     - ▬ Asymptomatic patients with risk factors
  2. If the 16MD-CTA is equivocal or if it is negative but the clinical suspicion remains high: a catheter arteriogram should be done (otherwise, if negative: stop).

Suggested Reading

Stokum JA, Gerzanich V, Simard JM. Molecular pathophysiology of cerebral edema. J Cereb Blood Flow Metab. 2016;36(3):513–38.

Colomer CB, Vergara FS, Perez FT, Vasquez FM, Kunstmann AH, Fierro GP, Zenkovich CS. Delayed intracranial hypertension and cerebral edema in severe pediatric head injury: risk factor analysis. Pediatr Neurosurg. 2012;48(4):205–9.

Liang D, Bhatta S, Gerzanich V, Simard JM. Cytotoxic edema: mechanisms of pathological cell swelling. Neurosurg Focus. 2007;22(5):1–9.

Barzó P, Marmarou A, Fatouros P, Hayasaki K, Corwin F. Contribution of vasogenic and cellular edema to traumatic brain swelling measured by diffusion-weighted imaging. J Neurosurg. 1997;87(6):900–7.

Fodstad H, Kelly PJ, Buchfelder M. History of the cushing reflex. Neurosurgery. 2006;59(5):1132–7.

Parizel PM, Makkat S, Jorens PG, Özsarlak Ö, Cras P, Van Goethem JW, Van Den Hauwe L, Verlooy J, De Schepper AM. Brainstem hemorrhage in descending transtentorial herniation (Duret hemorrhage). Intensive Care Med. 2002;28(1):85–8.

Kostecki K, Pearson-Shaver AL. Subfalcine Herniation. StatPearls [Internet], 2019.

Decker R, Pearson-Shaver AL. Uncal herniation. StatPearls [Internet], 2020.

Ishikawa M, Kikuchi H, Fujisawa I, Yonekawa Y. Tonsillar herniation on magnetic resonance imaging. Neurosurgery. 1988;22(1):77–81.

Cuneo RA, Caronna JJ, Pitts L, Townsend J, Winestock DP. Upward transtentorial herniation: seven cases and a literature review. Arch Neurol. 1979;36(10):618–23.

Chen JW, Gombart ZJ, Rogers S, Gardiner SK, Cecil S, Bullock RM. Pupillary reactivity as an early indicator of increased intracranial pressure: the introduction of the neurological pupil index. Surg Neurol Int. 2011;2:82.

Kanagalingam S, Miller NR. Horner syndrome: clinical perspectives. Eye Brain. 2015;7:35.

Clark A, Mesfin FB. Trauma neurological exam.

Pearce JM. Parinaud's syndrome. J Neurol Neurosurg Psychiatry. 2005;76(1):99.

North JB, Jennett S. Abnormal breathing patterns associated with acute brain damage. Arch Neurol. 1974;31(5):338–44.

Bricolo A, Turazzi S, Alexandre A, Rizzuto N. Decerebrate rigidity in acute head injury. J Neurosurg. 1977;47(5):680–98.

Goila AK, Pawar M. The diagnosis of brain death. Indian J Crit Care Med: peer-reviewed, official publication of Indian Society of Critical Care Medicine. 2009;13(1):7.

Simakurthy S, Tripathy K. Oculovestibular reflex. StatPearls [Internet], 2020.

Wang MY, Wallace P, Gruen JP. Brain death documentation: analysis and issues. Neurosurgery. 2002;51(3):731–6.

Brown CV, Zada G, Salim A, Inaba K, Kasotakis G, Hadjizacharia P, Demetriades D, Rhee P. Indications for routine repeat head computed tomography (CT) stratified by severity of traumatic brain injury. J Trauma Acute Care Surg. 2007;62(6):1339–45.

Ding J, Yuan F, Guo Y, Chen SW, Gao WW, Wang G, Cao HL, Ju SM, Chen H, Zhang PQ, Tian HL. A prospective clinical study of routine repeat computed tomography (CT) after traumatic brain injury (TBI). Brain Inj. 2012;26(10):1211–6.

Maas AI, Hukkelhoven CW, Marshall LF, Steyerberg EW. Prediction of outcome in traumatic brain injury with computed tomographic characteristics: a comparison between the computed tomographic classification and combinations of computed tomographic predictors. Neurosurgery. 2005;57(6):1173–82.

Deepika A, Prabhuraj AR, Saikia A, Shukla D. Comparison of predictability of Marshall and Rotterdam CT scan scoring system in determining early mortality after traumatic brain injury. Acta Neurochir. 2015;157(11):2033–8.

Marshall LF, Marshall SB, Klauber MR, Van Berkum CM, Eisenberg HO, Jane JA, Luerssen TG, Marmarou A, Foulkes MA. The diagnosis of head injury requires a classification based on computed axial tomography. J Neurotrauma. 1992;9(Suppl 1):S287–92.

Smith M. Multimodality neuromonitoring in adult traumatic brain injury: a narrative review. Anesthesiology. 2018;128(2):401–15.

Larach DB, Kofke WA, Le Roux P. Potential non-hypoxic/ischemic causes of increased cerebral interstitial fluid lactate/pyruvate ratio: a review of available literature. Neurocrit Care. 2011;15(3):609–22.

Carteron L, Bouzat P, Oddo M. Cerebral microdialysis monitoring to improve individualized neurointensive care therapy: an update of recent clinical data. Front Neurol. 2017;8:601.

Cormio M, Valadka AB, Robertson CS. Elevated jugular venous oxygen saturation after severe head injury. Neurosurg Focus. 2001;11(4):9–15.

Le Roux PD, Newell DW, Lam AM, Grady MS, Winn HR. Cerebral arteriovenous oxygen difference: a predictor of cerebral infarction and outcome in patients with severe head injury. J Neurosurg. 1997;87(1):1–8.

Armstead WM. Cerebral blood flow autoregulation and dysautoregulation. Anesthesiol Clin. 2016;34(3):465–77.

Bratton SL, Chestnut RM, Ghajar J, McConnell HFF, Harris OA, Hartl R, Manley GT, Nemecek A, Newell DW, Rosenthal G, Schouten J. VI. Indications for intracranial pressure monitoring. J Neurotrauma. 2007;24(Supplement 1):S-37.

Aiolfi A, Khor D, Cho J, Benjamin E, Inaba K, Demetriades D. Intracranial pressure monitoring in severe blunt head trauma: does the type of monitoring device matter? J Neurosurg. 2017;128(3):828–33.

Tavakoli S, Peitz G, Ares W, Hafeez S, Grandhi R. Complications of invasive intracranial pressure monitoring devices in neurocritical care. Neurosurg Focus. 2017;43(5):E6.

Aylward SC. Intracranial hypertension: is it primary, secondary, or idiopathic? J Neurosci Rural Pract. 2014;5(4):326.

Cardoso ER, Rowan JO, Galbraith S. Analysis of the cerebrospinal fluid pulse wave in intracranial pressure. J Neurosurg. 1983;59(5):817–21.

Hawthorne C, Piper I. Monitoring of intracranial pressure in patients with traumatic brain injury. Front Neurol. 2014;5:121.

Wijdicks EF. Lundberg and his waves. Neurocrit Care. 2019;31(3):546–9.

Cole CD, Gottfried ON, Liu JK, Couldwell WT. Hyponatremia in the neurosurgical patient: diagnosis and management. Neurosurg Focus. 2004;16(4):1–0.

Leonard J, Garrett RE, Salottolo K, Slone DS, Mains CW, Carrick MM, Bar-Or D. Cerebral salt wasting after traumatic brain injury: a review of the literature. Scand J Trauma Resusc Emerg Med. 2015;23(1):1–7.

Harrigan MR. Cerebral salt wasting syndrome: a review. Neurosurgery. 1996;38(1):152–60.

Sepehri P, Abbasi Z, Mohammadi NS, Bagheri S, Fattahian R. Hyponatremia in traumatic brain injury patients: Syndrome of Inappropriate Antidiuretic Hormone (SIADH) versus Cerebral Salt Wasting Syndrome (CSWS). J Inj Violence Res. 2012;4(3 Suppl 1):17.

Palmer BF. Hyponatraemia in a neurosurgical patient: syndrome of inappropriate antidiuretic hormone secretion versus cerebral salt wasting. Nephrol Dial Transpl. 2000;15(2):262–8.

Capatina C, Paluzzi A, Mitchell R, Karavitaki N. Diabetes insipidus after traumatic brain injury. J Clin Med. 2015;4(7):1448–62.

Kalra S, Zargar AH, Jain SM, Sethi B, Chowdhury S, Singh AK, Thomas N, Unnikrishnan AG, Thakkar PB, Malve H. Diabetes insipidus: the other diabetes. Indian J Endocrinol Metabol. 2016;20(1):9.

Alexiou GA, Sfakianos G, Prodromou N. Pediatric head trauma. J Emerg Trauma Shock. 2011;4(3):403.

Lee SJ, Kim JK, Kim SJ. The clinical characteristics and prognosis of subgaleal hemorrhage in newborn. Korean J Pediatr. 2018;61(12):387.

Choi J, Lee IW, Yang J, Lee HJ, Yeo IS, Yi JS, Lim JK. Chronic ossified subperiosteal hematoma of the skull in an 11-year-old child: a case report. Childs Nerv Syst. 2011;27(7):1165–8.

Singh I, Rohilla S, Siddiqui SA, Kumar P. Growing skull fractures: guidelines for early diagnosis and surgical management. Childs Nerv Syst. 2016;32(6):1117–22.

Wright JN. CNS injuries in abusive head trauma. Am J Roentgenol. 2017;208(5):991–1001.

Binenbaum G, Chen W, Huang J, Ying GS, Forbes BJ. The natural history of retinal hemorrhage in pediatric head trauma. J AAPOS. 2016;20(2):131–5.

Kazim SF, Shamim MS, Tahir MZ, Enam SA, Waheed S. Management of penetrating brain injury. J Emerg Trauma Shock. 2011;4(3):395.

Kazim SF, Shamim MS, Tahir MZ, Enam SA, Waheed S. Management of penetrating brain injury. J Emerg Trauma Shock. 2011;4(3):395.

Esnault P, Cardinale M, Boret H, D'Aranda E, Montcriol A, Bordes J, Prunet B, Joubert C, Dagain A, Goutorbe P, Kaiser E. Blunt cerebrovascular injuries in severe traumatic brain injury: incidence, risk factors, and evolution. J Neurosurg. 2016;127(1):16–22.

Miller PR, Fabian TC, Bee TK, Timmons S, Chamsuddin A, Finkle R, Croce MA. Blunt cerebrovascular injuries: diagnosis and treatment. J Trauma Acute Care Surg. 2001;51(2):279–86.

Rutman AM, Vranic JE, Mossa-Basha M. Imaging and management of blunt cerebrovascular injury. Radiographics. 2018;38(2):542–63.

Management of Cranial Neurotrauma

Abdullah H. Al Ramadan, Sarah A. Basindwah,
Silky Chotai, Mohammed A. Al-Rawi, Ahmed Nabil,
Alaa H. Arkawazi, Haitham A. Obaid,
Zahraa F. Al-Sharshahi, and Iype Cherian

Contents

Suggested Reading – 46

© The Author(s), under exclusive license to Springer Nature Switzerland AG 2022
S. S. Hoz et al., *Neurotrauma*, https://doi.org/10.1007/978-3-030-80869-3_2

2

❓ 1. Cushing's reflex?
The *FALSE* answer is:
A. It is a late sign of increased ICP.
B. It indicates that brainstem herniation is imminent.
C. Patients with two of three signs of the Cushing's reflex have been found to have almost two-fold higher mortality than patients with stable vital signs.
D. It is a triad of hypotension, bradycardia, and tachypnea.
E. Cushing's reflex can result in systemic vasoconstriction.

✅ Answer D
— Cushing's reflex is a physiological nervous system response to acute elevations of intracranial pressure (ICP) resulting in the Cushing triad of widened pulse pressure (increasing systolic, decreasing diastolic), bradycardia, and irregular respirations.

❓ 2. Indications for head CT scan in mild TBI
The *FALSE* answer is:
A. GCS less than 13 during initial assessment
B. History of loss of consciousness >5 min at the scene
C. History of prior TBI
D. Intoxicated patient
E. GCS less than 15 after resuscitation

✅ Answer C
— (A history of remote head trauma is not an indication for a head CT scan following a mild TBI).

❓ 3. Indications to perform a head CT scan within the first hour following TBI
The *FALSE* answer is:
A. GCS less than 13 on initial assessment
B. More than one episode of vomiting
C. Isolated posttraumatic seizure
D. Head injury on warfarin
E. Acute head injury with brief period of loss of consciousness and age >65 years

✅ Answer E
— According to the national institute for health and care excellence (NICE) guidelines for CT Head Scan in Patients Presenting with TBI,

the action required when the patient is age 65 years or older is CT head scan within 8 hour of head injury.

❓ 4. Indications for head CT in acute TBI, Canadian CT head rule,
   The *FALSE* answer is:
   A. The rule applies to the head-injured patients with GCS 13–15/15 and witnessed loss of consciousness, amnesia, or confusion.
   B. High-risk group includes those with GCS 13–15 and are aged 65 or older.
   C. Medium risk criteria include dangerous mechanism of head injury.
   D. Medium risk criteria include two or more episodes of vomiting.
   E. Medium risk criteria include >30 min retrograde amnesia.

✅ Answer D
   ▬ According to the Canadian CT Head Rule, CT head is mandatory if one or more of the following high-risk criteria for neurosurgical intervention are present: (1) GCS score less than 15 at 2 h after head injury; (2) suspected open or depressed skull fracture; (3) any sign of basal skull fracture (e.g. hemotympanum, "raccoon" eyes, CSF otorrhea/rhinorrhea, Battle's sign); (4) two or more episodes of vomiting; and (5) patient is 65 years of age or older.
   ▬ CT head is also recommended in patients in the medium-risk category who may have clinically important brain injuries that may require admission: (1) greater than 30 min of retrograde amnesia or (2) injury via a "dangerous mechanism" (e.g. motor vehicle accident versus pedestrian, ejection from motor vehicle, fall from greater than 3 feet or down five or more stairs).

❓ 5. Imaging in TBI,
   The *FALSE* answer is:
   A. CT scan is superior to MRI for diagnosing diffuse axial injury (DAI).
   B. CT is better for acute subdural hematoma (SDH) than magnetic resonance imaging (MRI).
   C. MRI is more sensitive than CT in identifying isodense SDH.
   D. Subarachnoid hemorrhage is seen better in CT than MRI.
   E. 40–50% of linear skull fractures can be missed on axial projection in CT.

2

✅ **Answer A**
- For diagnosing DAI, MRI is superior to CT scan. MRI brain without contrast is recommended for diagnosis of DAI. It is well delineated on gradient echo (GRE) sequence. Studies have demonstrated that the MRI does not alter the management or the outcomes. MRI is typically obtained for prognostication in cases of severe TBI.

❓ **6. Moderate TBI,**
The *FALSE* answer is:
A. GCS 9–12
B. 30% chance of having a brain lesion
C. 55% mortality
D. Loss of consciousness >30 min
E. Loss of consciousness <24 h

✅ **Answer C**
- The mortality rate in moderate TBI is around 15%. Moderate TBIs can present with mild symptoms that get worse overtime.

❓ **7. Neurogenic shock with TBI,**
The *FALSE* answer is:
A. Increased right atrial pressure
B. Normal or decreased pulmonary capillary wedge pressure
C. Increased cardiac index
D. Decreased systemic vascular resistance
E. Decreased venous capacitance

✅ **Answer C**
- Neurogenic shock is characterized by increased right atrial pressure, normal or decreased pulmonary capillary wedge pressure, decreased cardiac index, decreased systemic vascular resistance, and decreased venous capacitance.

❓ **8. Anti-convulsants in TBI,**
The *FALSE* answer is:
A. Decrease the incidence of late posttraumatic seizures
B. Recommended for a maximum of 1 week
C. Prophylaxis for late posttraumatic seizures is not recommended
D. Phenytoin is the first-line medication
E. Prophylaxis for mild and moderate TBI is not recommended

✅ **Answer A**
- Early posttraumatic seizures occur within the first week following TBI, while late seizures occur after the first week. Antiepileptic prophylaxis decreases the incidence of early posttraumatic seizures, but does not impact the occurrence of late posttraumatic seizures.

❓ **9. Steroids in TBI,**

The *FALSE* answer is:

A. Increase mortality
B. Increase systematic complications in adults
C. Has no effect on cerebral edema in pediatrics
D. Has no effect on ICP
E. Only recommended in severe TBI

✅ **Answer E**
- In TBI, steroids increase morbidity and mortality with no evidence of clinical or ICP improvement. They are not recommended in TBI.

❓ **10. Indications for ICP monitoring in TBI,**

The *FALSE* answer is:

A. GCS 3–8 with abnormal CT scan
B. GCS 9–11 with cerebral contusion, without surgical intervention
C. Concomitant severe chest trauma requiring deep sedation
D. Diffuse injury type II (Marshall CT classification)
E. Diffuse injury type III (Marshall CT classification)

✅ **Answer D**
- Diffuse injury II Marshall CT classification is NOT an indication for ICP monitoring, while diffuse injury III is an indication. Diffuse injury II (Marshall CT classification: basal cisterns remain visible, no high or mixed density lesions >25 cm^3, midline shift of 0–5 mm) is not an indication for placement of ICP monitor in TBI. Diffuse injury III (Marshall CT classification: basal cisterns are compressed or absent, no high or mixed density lesions >25 cm^3, midline shift of 0–5 mm, and brain swelling) is an indication for ICP monitor placement.

❓ **11. ICP Waves,**

The *FALSE* answer is:

A. Lundberg A correlates with decreased cerebral compliance.
B. Lundberg B is associated with respiratory fluctuations in PaCO2.

2

    C. Lundberg C is associated with systemic changes in arterial pressure.
    D. In case of hydrocephalus, the P2 wave disappears.
    E. If P2 amplitude exceeds P1 that indicates decreased compliance.

✅ **Answer D**
- P2 wave of ICP represents cerebral compliance. When the ventricular walls are stiffened by hydrocephalus and lack compliance, the P2 wave will increase with amplitude higher than P1.

❓ **12. ICP,**
    The *FALSE* answer is:
    A. In severe TBI, the cerebral perfusion pressure (CPP) goal is below 70.
    B. EVD chamber height of 10 mmHg indicates an ICP of 20 cm H_2O.
    C. The brain autoregulates the CPP to maintain a stable cerebral blood flow at 55–60 mL/100 g/min.
    D. Surgical management is reserved for refractory ICP.
    E. Autoregulation is lost in severe TBI.

✅ **Answer B**
- An EVD flow chamber height 1 mmHg indicates an ICP of 1.36 cm H_2O.

❓ **13. Management of elevated ICP,**
    The *FALSE* answer is:
    A. Hyperventilation is not recommended during the first 24 hours.
    B. Hyperventilation can decrease ICP by decreasing pH.
    C. There is a 2% decrease in cerebral blood flow for every 1 mmHg decrease in PaCO2.
    D. Inducing moderate hypercapnia up to 30 mmHg is recommended.
    E. PaCO2 levels below 25 mmHg can cause cerebral ischemia.

✅ **Answer B**
- Hyperventilation decreases the ICP by increasing the pH.

❓ **14. Mechanism of barbiturate-induced coma,**
    The *FALSE* answer is:
    A. Decreased extracellular concentration of lactate
    B. Decreased excitatory amino acids

C. Decreased cerebral oxygen requirement
D. Activation of free radical lipid peroxidation
E. Prophylactic use associated with worse outcome

✅ **Answer D**
- The mechanism of barbiturate-induced coma is "inverse steal phenomenon." They act by inhibition of free radical lipid peroxidation.

❓ **15. Phenobarbital use in raised ICP,**
   The *FALSE* answer is:
   A. Pentobarbital is a last tier therapy for medical management of raised ICP.
   B. It provides maximal reduction in cerebral oxygen requirements and blood flow.
   C. Brain death examination can be conducted at 8 h following phenobarbital use.
   D. Should be titrated to burst suppression on EEG.
   E. Vitals should be monitored for hypotension.

✅ **Answer C**
- Phenobarbital can confound any attempts of brain death examination until it has been completely metabolized from the system, which can take days. High-dose barbiturate administration is recommended to control refractory ICP.

❓ **16. Mannitol use in TBI,**
   The *FALSE* answer is:
   A. The recommended dose is 0.5 gm/kg to 1 gm/kg.
   B. Serum osmolality should not exceed 320 mosmol/L.
   C. Long-term use is recommended for severe TBI.
   D. It has a neuroprotective role by scavangaing free radicals.
   E. Increases blood-brain barrier permeability.

✅ **Answer C**
- Long-term use of mannitol is not recommended in TBI, as it may result in dilutional hyponatremia, acute renal failure, and disruption of blood–brain barrier.

2

? **17. Hypothermia in TBI,**
   The *FALSE* answer is:
   A. Therapeutic hypothermia should be initiated within the first 24 h.
   B. Therapeutic hypothermia should be titrated according to the ICP.
   C. Prophylactic hypothermia improves outcomes.
   D. The goal temperature is 33–35 °C.
   E. Permissive hyperthermia may exacerbate brain damage.

✓ **Answer C**
   ▬ There is no evidence suggesting that prophylactic hypothermia in TBI patients leads to better outcomes.

? **18. ICU management in severe TBI,**
   The *FALSE* answer is:
   A. Feeding could be initiated by the seventh day post injury, at most.
   B. Transgastric jejunal feeding is associated with reduced incidence of ventilator-associated pneumonia.
   C. Early tracheostomy reduces the incidence of nosocomial pneumonia.
   D. Povidone–iodine oral care is not recommended to reduce ventilator-associated pneumonia.
   E. Povidone–iodine oral care increases the risk of acute respiratory distress syndrome.

✓ **Answer C**
   ▬ There is no evidence that early tracheostomy reduces mortality or the rate of nosocomial pneumonia. Feeding patients to attain basal caloric replacement as early as fifth day latest by the seventh day post-injury is recommended to decrease mortality.

? **19. Scalp lacerations management,**
   The *FALSE* answer is:
   A. Tight head bandage can efficiently control scalp bleeding.
   B. It is best managed with rapid closure of the skin with staples.
   C. Raney clips may be helpful for temporary closure.
   D. There is no need for separate galeal closure.
   E. Monitoring vitals for systemic hypotension is needed.

✅ **Answer A**
- Scalp lacerations can result in exsanguination. Definitive stapling is needed to stop the bleeding.

❓ **20. Depressed skull fractures,**
The *FALSE* answer is:
A. Inner table fractures are depressed.
B. CT is mandatory to exclude depressed fractures.
C. Prophylactic antibiotics are indicated for closed depressed fractures.
D. Evidence of dural penetration is an indication for surgery.
E. Water-tight dural closure is required.

✅ **Answer C**
- Patients with open depressed skull fractures may benefit from prophylactic antibiotics. Physical examination of the fracture is not sufficient to exclude depressed skull fracture, and a CT scan is mandatory. The presence of clinical or radiological evidence of dural penetration is an indication for surgical intervention. Surgical management consists of bony elevation, debridement, and watertight dural closure.

❓ **21. Traumatic CSF leaks,**
The *FALSE* answer is:
A. Most leaks are managed conservatively.
B. Pneumococcal vaccine is indicated.
C. Acetazolamide is a treatment option.
D. Serial lumbar puncture is one of the conservative options.
E. B1-transferrin is the bedside diagnostic test of choice.

✅ **Answer E**
- Most traumatic CSF leaks resolve within a week and only require observation (bed rest, (avoidance of any straining maneuvers), pneumococcal vaccine). The exact site of the leak can be detected with a CT and water-soluble intrathecal contrast.

❓ **22. Traumatic CSF leaks,**
The *FALSE* answer is:
A. Prophylactic antibiotics are indicated.
B. Primary repair is indicated for copious leaks

2

C. Primary repair is indicated for leaks that persist for 7 days.
D. Skull-base reconstruction is one of the surgical options.
E. Musculo-fascial flap is one of the surgical options.

✔️ **Answer A**
- Prophylactic antibiotics do not prevent meningitis and increase the risk of developing resistant organisms.

❓ **23. Traumatic facial palsy,**
The *FALSE* answer is:
A. Steroids are used for delayed-onset facial paresis.
B. Otic capsule sparing fractures result in facial palsy.
C. Otic capsule sparing fractures are explored by the translabyrinthine approach.
D. Facial nerve injury commonly occurs at the perigeniculate region
E. Supralabyrinthine approach spares sensorineural hearing function.

✔️ **Answer B**
- Injuries involving the otic capsule with loss of hearing are explored by a translabyrinthine approach. In well-aerated mastoid air cells or with ossicular discontinuity, a transmastoid/supralabyrinthine approach is used. In poorly aerated mastoid air cells or when a severe facial nerve is encountered in the supralabyrinthine approach, a combined transmastoid/middle cranial fossa technique is used. Facial nerve injury commonly occurs at the perigeniculate region and mastoid segment. Immediate onset, incomplete traumatic facial palsies do not usually require surgical exploration.

❓ **24. Tension pneumocephalus, management,**
The *FALSE* answer is:
A. Drain CSF from a pre-existing EVD
B. Burr hole decompression
C. Cranialization of the frontal sinus
D. Decompressive craniectomy
E. Place EVD for aspiration of air

✔️ **Answer A**
- Draining CSF in the setting of possible tension pneumocephalus is contraindicated.

? 25. Epidural hematoma (EDH),
   The *FALSE* answer is:
   A. The lucid interval phenomenon occurs in more than half of cases.
   B. Dilatation of ipsilateral pupil occurs in less than half of cases.
   C. Decreased level of consciousness is a common presentation.
   D. It carries excellent surgical prognosis.
   E. Posterior fossa EDH has better outcome in children.

✓ Answer A
   ▬ The lucid interval phenomena occur in 14–21% of EDH cases.

? 26. Epidural hematoma,
   The *FALSE* answer is:
   A. Hypodensity on CT within an EDH is associated with worse prognosis.
   B. Ratio of female:male = 4:1.
   C. Rare before age 2 or after age 60.
   D. 90% associated with skull fracture.
   E. EDH is less common in children.

✓ Answer B
   ▬ Ratio of male:female = 4:1.

? 27. Venous epidural hematoma,
   The *FALSE* answer is:
   A. Half of EDH cases are due to venous bleeding.
   B. Occurs due to laceration of sphenoparietal sinus.
   C. Occurs due to fracture of the greater sphenoid wing.
   D. Venous EDH more commonly occurs in the absence of skull fracture.
   E. Venous EDH is often benign in nature.

✓ Answer A
   ▬ Approximately 10% of EDHs are due to venous bleeding.

? 28. Epidural hematoma, surgical indications,
   The *FALSE* answer is:
   A. Volume <30 cm^3 with anisocoria and 20 mm maximal thickness
   B. Volume >30 cm^3

2

C. GCS 8 or less with evidence of anisocoria
D. Volume 15 cm^3 with >5 mm midline shift
E. Volume 20 cm^3 with GCS 10 without midline shift

✅ **Answer E**

— An EDH with a volume of less than 30 mls, thickness less than 15 mm, and a midline shift of less than 5 mm in patients with a GCS score greater than 8 without focal deficit can be managed nonoperatively with serial computed tomographic (CT) scans and close neurological observation in a neurosurgical center. Location is an important factor in the surgical decision. Large or expanding temporal hematomas may lead to uncal herniation and rapid deterioration. EDH in the posterior fossa often requires prompt evacuation due to the limited space available.

❓ **29. Subdural hematoma (SDH),**
The *FALSE* answer is:
A. Most commonly due to tearing of cortical bridging veins
B. May occur due to disruption of superficial cerebral arteries
C. Crosses suture lines
D. More commonly located at the coup site
E. Calcification occurs in up to 3% of chronic hematomas

✅ **Answer D**

— Unlike EDH, SDH is more often located at the countercoup site.

❓ **30. Subdural hematoma,**
The *FALSE* answer is:
A. The most common focal traumatic intracranial lesion.
B. Acute SDH is defined within 24 h of injury.
C. 10% of acute SDH will appear as isodense in non-contrasted CT brain.
D. The thickness of the hematoma has a prognostic value.
E. Age is a major factor influencing mortality.

✅ **Answer B**

— Acute SDH is defined within 72 h of insult.

❓ 31. Acute subdural hematoma,
The *FALSE* answer is:
A. Thickness greater than 10 mm is an indication for surgery.
B. Midline shift greater than 5 mm is an indication for surgery.
C. GCS score less than 9 is in itself an indication for surgery.
D. GCS drop by two or more points since injury is an indication for surgery.
E. GCS score less than 9 is an indication for ICP monitoring.

✓ Answer C
➖ A comatose patient (GCS score less than 9) with a SDH less than 10 mm thick and a midline shift less than 5 mm should undergo surgical evacuation if the GCS score dropped by two or more points between the time of injury and hospital admission and/or the patient presents with asymmetric or fixed and dilated pupils and/or the ICP exceeds 20 mmHg.

❓ 32. Traumatic subarachnoid hemorrhage,
The *FALSE* answer is:
A. Commonly seen immediately adjacent to brain contusions
B. Not commonly seen in the Sylvian fissure
C. Usually seen in the basal cisterns
D. Often seen in the peripheral cerebral sulci
E. Isolated traumatic SAH is best managed conservatively

✓ Answer C
➖ Traumatic SAH is usually located on the cerebral convexity rather than the cisterns.

❓ 33. Traumatic intraparenchymal or intracerebral hemorrhage (ICH),
The *FALSE* answer is:
A. Smaller lesions do not require surgical evacuation.
B. Cerebellar ICH >3 cm should be managed operatively.
C. GCS 6–8 with temporal contusions and cisternal compression should be treated operatively.
D. All lesions >50 cm^3 should be treated palliatively.
E. ICH with no mass effect should be managed conservatively.

2

✅ **Answer D**
- Patients with intraparenchymal lesions greater than 50 cm³ in volume should be treated operatively. The decision of palliative care should take in to account multiple parameters including but not limited to patients' comorbidities, clinical exam, GCS, and CT scan findings.

❓ **34. Traumatic intraventricular hemorrhage (IVH),**
The *FALSE* answer is:
A. Tearing of subependymal vessels
B. Due to retrograde reflux of SAH
C. Up to 5% of closed head injury
D. Extension of intraparenchymal hemorrhage
E. The third ventricle is the most common site

✅ **Answer E**
- Traumatic IVH is most commonly seen in the lateral ventricles (occipital horns).

❓ **35. Penetrating traumatic brain injury,**
The *FALSE* answer is:
A. Broad spectrum antibiotics are indicated.
B. Anti-seizure medications are indicated.
C. Open surgical debridement is indicated.
D. Antibiotics are not indicated after removal of foreign body.
E. Foreign body removal only to be done in the operating room.

✅ **Answer D**
- Empirical antibiotics are indicated before and after removal of the foreign body.

❓ **36. Penetrating TBI-associated vascular injury,**
The *FALSE* answer is:
A. Increases with frontal injury
B. Increases with orbito-craniocerebral injury
C. Increases with occipital injury
D. Increases with trans-basal injury
E. Found in 30% of penetrating TBI treated by decompressive craniectomy

✅ **Answer C**
- The risk of vascular injury is lower with occipital injury compared to other intracranial injuries.

❓ **37. Penetrating TBI, poor prognostic factors,**
The *FALSE* answer is:
A. Involvement of air sinuses
B. Involvement of multiple lobes
C. IVH
D. Crosses the midline
E. Perforating type of injury

✅ **Answer A**
- Involvement of the air sinuses or mastoid air cells increases the chances of CSF leak and meningitis, but is not associated with poor prognosis in the setting of penetrating TBI.

❓ **38. Penetrating TBI,**
The *FALSE* answer is:
A. Craniectomy is indicated for debridement of contused brain
B. Accessible missile fragments should be removed.
C. Wound irrigation should be performed.
D. Bedside laceration repair has the best prognosis.
E. No need to remove deep-seated sharpnel.

✅ **Answer D**
- There are reports of either superficial only (local irrigation and wound closure) or aggressive approaches (craniotomy and thorough debridement of injured brain and the gun shot tract for removal of deep fragments) to treatment. However, the best evidence supports an intermediate approach.

❓ **39. Nonaccidental pediatric TBI,**
The *FALSE* answer is:
A. One-third of cases missed at the initial presentation.
B. One-third of cases have retinal hemorrhage.
C. Acute subdural hematoma is the most common associated hemorrhage.

2

D. The most common history is no history of trauma.
E. Bilateral diffuse hypodensity on CT associated with poor outcome.

✅ **Answer B**
– Retinal hemorrhage is present in, at least two-thirds of the cases. Additional social work investigation and ophthalmology consult are warranted in nonaccidental trauma.

❓ **40. Pediatric ping-pong skull fractures,**
The *FALSE* answer is:
A. If neurologically intact, observation is recommended.
B. Follow up CT is needed to ensure proper healing.
C. Bulging around the fracture site can indicate dural tear.
D. Progressive widening of the fracture is an indication for craniotomy.
E. High ICP is the main indication for surgery.

✅ **Answer E**
– In a neurologically normal infant, this fracture should be managed nonoperatively. This is the classic "ping-pong" fracture, and over time the CSF pulsations will remodel the bone and heal this fracture. Operative intervention is generally not required. Cosmetic outcome is the main indication for surgery.
– In case of fracture widening on follow-up, a circumferential craniotomy and dural repair are needed.

❓ **41. TBI-related complications,**
The *FALSE* answer is:
A. Disseminated intravascular coagulation (DIC)
B. Highest rate of hematoma detection is in the second week of TBI
C. Infection is more common with low-velocity penetrating injury
D. 10% risk of infection despite the use of prophylactic antibiotics
E. Up to 40% have early onset seizures in severe TBI

✅ **Answer B**
– The highest rate of intracranial hematoma detection is at 3–8 h after initial injury. Disseminated intravascular coagulation (DIC) after TBI due to release of thromboplastin from damaged brain tissue.

? **42. TBI-related retroclival hematoma,**
  The *FALSE* answer is:
  A. More common in children
  B. Caused by disruption of the tectorial membrane
  C. Caused by bleeding from the basilar venous plexus
  D. Atlanto-axial disruption should be excluded
  E. Not seen in head CT

✓ **Answer E**
  ▬ It can be seen on head CT. Atlanto-occipital or atlanto-axial disruption should be excluded.

? **43. Cephalohematoma,**
  The *FALSE* answer is:
  A. Most do not require surgical intervention
  B. Head wrapping is a treatment option
  C. Needle aspiration is the treatment of choice
  D. Blood investigation to check for anemia
  E. The bulge may take 7 days to resolve

✓ **Answer C**
  ▬ Cephalhematoma resolves spontaneously. It may be treated with head wrapping to accelerate the resolution. Needle aspiration is used very rarely for special cases with very large hematoma.

? **44. Concussion,**
  The *FALSE* answer is:
  A. Headache is the most common symptom
  B. Linked to an increase release of glutamate
  C. Consciousness is preserved in up to 90% of cases
  D. Retrograde and anterograde amnesia can occur
  E. Aspirin is the treatment of choice

✓ **Answer E**
  ▬ Aspirin and other NSAIDs should be avoided for post-concussion headache in the acute period.

2

❓ 45. DAI (diffuse axonal injury),

The *FALSE* answer is:

A. Diagnosis confirmed by immunostaining for B-amyloid precursor protein

B. Susceptibility-weighted imaging is more sensitive than MRI FLAIR sequence

C. Traumatic loss of consciousness less than 6 h considered as mild DAI

D. Moderate DAI is not associated with decerebrate posturing

E. Severe DAI is associated with 50% mortality

✅ Answer C

- Traumatic loss of consciousness less than 6 h considered as concussion.
- Mild DAI: Coma of 6–24 h
- Moderate DAI: Come of more than 24 h
- Severe DAI: Moderate + decerebrate posturing or flaccidity

❓ 46. TBI markers,

The *FALSE* answer is:

A. GFAP is associated with acute TBI

B. GFAP can determine the need to undergo CT scan

C. Tau proteins are an indicator for glial injury

D. S100B can demonstrate glial injury

E. "TBI" markers may be false positive in cases of polytrauma

✅ Answer C

- Markers like UCH- L1, neuron-specific enolase (NSE), and proteins (Tau) demonstrate neuronal injury.

❓ 47. TBI, Marshal classification,

The *FALSE* answer is:

A. Type I has normal CT brain.

B. Midline shift is not included in type II.

C. Type III has no cisternal compression.

D. Type IV is the most fatal type.

E. Type V denoted surgically evacuated lesions.

✅ **Answer C**

- Marshal Classification is a CT scan-based grading used to predict the outcome in TBI. Type II associated with abnormal CT brain without compression of brainstem cisterns which associated with type III. More than 5-mm midline shift associated with type IV.

Marshall scoring of TBI			
	MLS[a]	Cisterns	High- or mixed-density lesion	Notes
I	None	Present	None	No visible pathology on CT scan
II	0–5 mm	Present	None	
III	0–5 mm	Compressed or absent	None	Swelling
IV	>5 mm		None	
V	Any	Any	Any	Any lesion surgically evacuate
VI			>25 cm^3	Not surgically evacuate

[a]MLS-midline shift

❓ **48. TBI, secondary injury,**
   The *FALSE* answer is:
   A. Hypoxia
   B. Axonal shearing
   C. Hyperglycemia
   D. Brain edema
   E. Vasospasm

✅ **Answer B**

- Primary TBI is the damage (more or less complete) caused by the trauma itself during the initial impact, like contusion, damage to blood vessels, and axonal shearing. Secondary Brain injury is injury due to the physiological response of the body to the primary TBI.
- Hypoperfusion with cerebral blood flow less than 33 mL/100 g per minute is associated with worse outcome. Traumatic SAH is an independent predictor of worse clinical outcome, and it is the most likely cause of delayed-onset posttraumatic vasospasm.

2

❓ 49. Glasgow Outcome Scale (GOS)?

The *FALSE* answer is:

A. Used for assessment of neurological outcome
B. Score of 5 indicates death
C. Score of 3 indicates severe disability
D. Score of 2 indicates persistent vegetative state
E. Lower and upper moderate disabilities are not part of the scale

✅ Answer B

━ GOS is a global scale for functional outcome that rates the patients' functional status into one of the five categories: Dead, Vegetative state, Severe disability, Moderate disability, and Good Recovery. The score of 5 on GOS indicates good outcome.

Summary	Glasgow Outcome Scale	Extended GOS
–	1: Dead	1: Dead
Sleep/awake	2: Persistent Vegetative State	2: Persistent Vegetative State
Conscious but dependent	3: Severe Disability	3: Lower Severe Disability 4: Upper Severe Disability
Independent but disabled	4: Moderate Disability	5: Lower Moderate Disability 6: Upper Moderate Disability
May have mild residual effects	5: Good Recovery	7: Lower Good Recovery 8: Upper Good Recovery

Suggested Reading

Agrawal D, Cochrane DD. Traumatic retroclival epidural hematoma—a pediatric entity? Childs Nerv Syst. 2006;22(7):670–3.

Almulhim AM, Madadin M. Scalp laceration. In: StatPearls [Internet]. Treasure Island: StatPearls Publishing; 2021.

Asfora WT, Schwebach L. A modified technique to treat chronic and subacute subdural hematoma. Surg Neurol. 2003;59(4):329–32.

Atzema C, Mower WR, Hoffman JR, Holmes JF, Killian AJ, Wolfson AB, National Emergency X-Radiography Utilization Study (NEXUS) II Group. Prevalence and prognosis of traumatic intraventricular hemorrhage in patients with blunt head trauma. J Trauma Acute Care Surg. 2006;60(5):1010–7.

Biersteker HA, Andriessen TM, Horn J, Franschman G, van der Naalt J, Hoedemaekers CW, Lingsma HF, Haitsma I, Vos PE. Factors influencing intracranial pressure monitoring guideline compliance and outcome after severe traumatic brain injury. Crit Care Med. 2012;40(6):1914–22.

Bodanapally UK, Saksobhavivat N, Shanmuganathan K, Aarabi B, Roy AK. Arterial injuries after penetrating brain injury in civilians: risk factors on admission head computed tomography. J Neurosurg. 2015;122(1):219–26.

Bramlett HM, Dietrich WD. Long-term consequences of traumatic brain injury: current status of potential mechanisms of injury and neurological outcomes. J Neurotrauma. 2015;32(23):1834–48.

Brown CV, Zada G, Salim A, Inaba K, Kasotakis G, Hadjizacharia P, Demetriades D, Rhee P. Indications for routine repeat head computed tomography (CT) stratified by severity of traumatic brain injury. J Trauma Acute Care Surg. 2007;62(6):1339–45.

Brown AW, Pretz CR, Bell KR, Hammond FM, Arciniegas DB, Bodien YG, Dams-O'Connor K, Giacino JT, Hart T, Johnson-Greene D, Kowalski RG. Predictive utility of an adapted Marshall head CT classification scheme after traumatic brain injury. Brain Inj. 2019;33(5):610–7.

Bullock MR, Chesnut R, Ghajar J, Gordon D, Hartl R, Newell DW, Servadei F, Walters BC, Wilberger J. Surgical management of depressed cranial fractures. Neurosurgery. 2006;58(suppl_3):S2–56.

Chang EF, Meeker M, Holland MC. Acute traumatic intraparenchymal hemorrhage: risk factors for progression in the early post-injury period. Neurosurgery. 2006;58(4):647–56.

Chesnut RM, Marshall LF, Klauber MR, Blunt BA, Baldwin N, Eisenberg HM, Jane JA, Marmarou A, Foulkes MA. The role of secondary brain injury in determining outcome from severe head injury. J Trauma Acute Care Surg. 1993;34(2):216–22.

Chesnut RM, Gautille T, Blunt BA, Klauber MR, Marshall LF. Neurogenic hypotension in patients with severe head injuries. J Trauma Acute Care Surg. 1998;44(6):958–63.

Cho SM, Kilic A, Dodd-o JM. Incomplete Cushing's reflex in extracorporeal membrane oxygenation. Int J Artif Organs. 2020;43(6):401–4.

Eftekhar B, Ghodsi M, Hadadi A, Taghipoor M, Sigarchi SZ, Rahimi-Movaghar V, Kazemzadeh ES, Esmaeeli B, Nejat F, Yalda A, Ketabchi E. Prophylactic antibiotic for prevention of posttraumatic meningitis after traumatic pneumocephalus: design and rationale of a placebo-controlled randomized multicenter trial [ISRCTN71132784]. Trials. 2006;7(1):1–4.

Fantacci F, Capozz D, Romano V, Ferrara P, Chiaretti A, Massimi L. "Spontaneous" ping-pong fracture in newborns: case report and review of the literature. Signa Vitae. 2015;10(1):103–9.

Fournier N, Gariepy C, Prévost JF, Belhumeur V, Fortier É, Carmichael PH, Gariepy JL, Le Sage N, Émond M. Adapting the Canadian CT head rule age criteria for mild traumatic brain injury. Emerg Med J. 2019;36(10):617–9.

Freeman WD. Erratum: management of intracranial pressure. Continuum (Minneap Minn). 2015;21(6):1550.

Geddes JF, Vowles GH, Beer TW, Ellison DW. The diagnosis of diffuse axonal injury: implications for forensic practice. Neuropathol Appl Neurobiol. 1997;23(4):339–47.

Gerber P, Coffman K. Nonaccidental head trauma in infants. Childs Nerv Syst. 2007;23(5):499–507.

2

Hernandez TD. Preventing post-traumatic epilepsy after brain injury: weighing the costs and benefits of anticonvulsant prophylaxis. Trends Pharmacol Sci. 1997;18(2):59–62.

Irie F, Le Brocque R, Kenardy J, Bellamy N, Tetsworth K, Pollard C. Epidemiology of traumatic epidural hematoma in young age. J Trauma Acute Care Surg. 2011;71(4):847–53.

Kazim SF, Shamim MS, Tahir MZ, Enam SA, Waheed S. Management of penetrating brain injury. J Emerg Trauma Shock. 2011;4(3):395.

Khairat A, Waseem M. Epidural hematoma. StatPearls; 2020.

King JT Jr, Carlier PM, Marion DW. Early Glasgow Outcome Scale scores predict long-term functional outcome in patients with severe traumatic brain injury. J Neurotrauma. 2005;22(9):947–54.

Laker SR. Epidemiology of concussion and mild traumatic brain injury. PM & R. 2011;3:S354–8.

Lee AL. Advanced imaging of traumatic brain injury. Korean J Neurotrauma. 2020;16(1):3.

LEE MW, DEPPE SA, SIPPERLY ME, BARRETTE RR, THOMPSON DR. The efficacy of barbiturate coma in the management of uncontrolled intracranial hypertension following neurosurgical trauma. J Neurotrauma. 1994;11(3):325–31.

Ling GS, Marshall SA. Management of traumatic brain injury in the intensive care unit. Neurol Clin. 2008a;26(2):409–26.

Ling GS, Marshall SA. Management of traumatic brain injury in the intensive care unit. Neurol Clin. 2008b;26(2):409–26.

Maugeri R, Anderson DG, Graziano F, Meccio F, Visocchi M, Iacopino DG. Conservative vs. surgical management of post-traumatic epidural hematoma: a case and review of literature. Am J Case Rep. 2015;16:811.

Nicholson L. Caput succedaneum and cephalohematoma: the cs that leave bumps on the head. Neonatal Netw. 2007;26(5):277–81.

Oh JW, Kim SH, Whang K. Traumatic cerebrospinal fluid leak: diagnosis and management. Korean J Neurotrauma. 2017;13(2):63.

Quaranta GC, Piazza F, Quaranta N, Ignazio Salonna A. Facial nerve paralysis in temporal bone fractures: outcomes after late decompression surgery. Acta Otolaryngol. 2001;121(5):652–5.

Robinson RG. Chronic subdural hematoma: surgical management in 133 patients. J Neurosurg. 1984;61(2):263–8.

Rondina C, Videtta W, Petroni G, Lujan S, Schoon P, Mori LB, Matkovich J, Carney N, Chesnut R. Mortality and morbidity from moderate to severe traumatic brain injury in Argentina. J Head Trauma Rehabil. 2005;20(4):368–76.

Rosenfeld JV, Bell RS, Armonda R. Current concepts in penetrating and blast injury to the central nervous system. World J Surg. 2015;39(6):1352–62.

Rubiano AM, Sanchez AI, Estebanez G, Peitzman A, Sperry J, Puyana JC. The effect of admission spontaneous hypothermia on patients with severe traumatic brain injury. Injury. 2013;44(9):1219–25.

Schwartz ML, Tator CH, Rowed DW, Reid SR, Meguro K, Andrews DF. The University of Toronto head injury treatment study: a prospective, randomized comparison of pentobarbital and mannitol. Can J Neurol Sci. 1984;11(4):434–40.

Seelig JM, Marshall LF, Toutant SM, Toole BM, Klauber MR, Bowers SA, Varnell JA. Traumatic acute epidural hematoma: unrecognized high lethality in comatose patients. Neurosurgery. 1984;15(5):617–20.

Shahrokhi N, Khaksari M, Soltani Z, Mahmoodi M, Nakhaee N. Effect of sex steroid hormones on brain edema, intracranial pressure, and neurologic outcomes after traumatic brain injury. Can J Physiol Pharmacol. 2010;88(4):414–21.

Siman R, Toraskar N, Dang A, McNeil E, McGarvey M, Plaum J, Maloney E, Grady MS. A panel of neuron-enriched proteins as markers for traumatic brain injury in humans. J Neurotrauma. 2009;26(11):1867–77.

Smith MC, Riskin BJ. The clinical use of barbiturates in neurological disorders. Drugs. 1991;42(3):365–78.

Stein SC, Burnett MG, Glick HA. Indications for CT scanning in mild traumatic brain injury: a cost-effectiveness study. J Trauma Acute Care Surg. 2006;61(3):558–66.

Tang A, Pandit V, Fennell V, Jones T, Joseph B, O'Keeffe T, Friese RS, Rhee P. Intracranial pressure monitor in patients with traumatic brain injury. J Surg Res. 2015;194(2):565–70.

Van Wyck DW, Grant GA, Laskowitz DT. Penetrating traumatic brain injury: a review of current evaluation and management concepts. J Neurol Neurophysiol. 2015;6(6):336–43.

Wilberger JE, Harris M, Diamond DL. Acute subdural hematoma: morbidity, mortality, and operative timing. J Neurosurg. 1991;74(2):212–8.

Wu Z, Li S, Lei J, An D, Haacke EM. Evaluation of traumatic subarachnoid hemorrhage using susceptibility-weighted imaging. Am J Neuroradiol. 2010;31(7):1302–10.

Yates H, Hamill M, Borel CO, Toung TJ. Incidence and perioperative management of tension pneumocephalus following craniofacial resection. J Neurosurg Anesthesiol. 1994;6(1):15–20.

Ziai WC, Torbey MT, Naff NJ, Williams MA, Bullock R, Marmarou A, Tuhrim S, Schmutzhard E, Pfausler B, Hanley DF. Frequency of sustained intracranial pressure elevation during treatment of severe intraventricular hemorrhage. Cerebrovasc Dis. 2009;27(4):403–10.

Complications, Outcome, and Other Aspects

Baha'eddin A. Muhsen, Bilal Ibrahim, Maria Laura Laffitte, Ignatius N. Esene, Hayder R. Salih, Zahraa F. Al-Sharshahi, and Iype Cherian

Contents

Suggested Reading – 61

© The Author(s), under exclusive license to Springer Nature Switzerland AG 2022
S. S. Hoz et al., *Neurotrauma*, https://doi.org/10.1007/978-3-030-80869-3_3

3

❓ 1. TBI-Seizures

The *FALSE* answer is:

A. Anticonvulsants prevent late-onset seizures.
B. Admission GCS is a strong risk factor for seizures.
C. Retained bone fragments are not significantly linked to post-traumatic epilepsy.
D. Penetrating brain injury has higher risk for epilepsy than closed TBI.
E. Antiepileptic prophylaxis is recommended only in the first week.

✔ Answer A

— Anticonvulsant prophylaxis has not been shown to prevent late-onset post-traumatic seizures.

❓ 2. TBI-Seizures

The *FALSE* answer is:

A. Posttraumatic epilepsy is recurrent seizures exceeding 7 days post-TBI.
B. Levetiracetam is recommended over phenytoin for early post-TBI seizures.
C. Subclinical post-TBI seizures rate is higher compared to clinical seizures.
D. Age >65 years is a risk factor for posttraumatic epilepsy.
E. ICH is a risk factor for both early and late post-TBI seizures.

✔ Answer B

— Levetiracetam is associated with increased frequency of abnormal EEG findings.

❓ 3. TBI-CSF leak

The *FALSE* answer is:

A. Trauma is the most common cause of CSF leak
B. Rhinorrhea is more common than otorrhea
C. 10-fold increase in overall infection rate
D. Meningitis incidence is 50%
E. 70–85% cease spontaneously by 2 weeks

✔ Answer D

— Meningitis incidence is 5–10%.

❓ 4. TBI-CSF leak

The *FALSE* answer is:
A. 1–3% of closed TBI.
B. TBI is the cause of 90% of cases in adults.
C. Middle fossa fractures have higher risk of leak than anterior fossa.
D. Temporal bone fractures can cause otorrhea or rhinorrhea.
E. Meningitis mortality rate secondary to posttraumatic CSF leak is about 10%.

✅ Answer C

▬ Anterior cranial fossa fractures have higher risk for CSF leak because the bone is thinner than the rest of the skull base and midline structures lack or have minimal dural investment.

❓ 5. TBI-CSF leak

The *FALSE* answer is:
A. 70% resolve within the first week.
B. Temporal bone fractures have the highest rate of spontaneous resolution.
C. Prophylactic antibiotics are not indicated in early leaks.
D. Lumbar drainage has high success rate for leak sealing.
E. Conservative management should continue for 2 weeks before considering surgery.

✅ Answer E

▬ Evidence indicates that CSF leakage that persists for >7 days has higher rate of meningitis. Conservative therapy should not continue more than 7 days, unless the patient's condition contraindicates surgery.

❓ 6. TBI-CSF leak

The *FALSE* answer is:
A. 50% present within the first 48 hours of TBI.
B. The cribriform plate fracture is the most common source of rhinorrhea.
C. The two most common complications of CSF fistulas are meningitis and pneumoencephalus.
D. Pneumoencephalon is pathognomic of skull base fracture.
E. Beta 2 transferrin is the gold standard to confirm CSF leak.

3

✅ **Answer B**

- The most common fracture sites leading to CSF rhinorrhea after TBI are the frontal sinus (30.8%), sphenoid sinus (11.4–30.8%), ethmoid sinus (15.4–19,1%), cribiform plate (7.7%), frontoethmoid (7.7%), and sphenoethmoid 7.7%.

❓ **7. TBI-Nutritional Support**
The *FALSE* answer is:
A. Energy expenditure up to 200% of normal
B. Nutritional supplementation within the first 72 hours
C. Early enteral feeding associated with lower mortality
D. Enteral feeding has lower risk of septicemia compared to parenteral route
E. Delayed gastric emptying precludes the enteral route of feeding

✅ **Answer E**

- Delayed gastric emptying does not preclude enteral feeding. If so, feeding via jejunal tube is usually successful.

❓ **8. TBI-Encephalopathy**
The *FALSE* answer is:
A. Symptoms onset at 40 years of age
B. Headache is a late manifestation
C. The severity of cognitive impairment is related to the amount of tau protein
D. Generalized cerebral atrophy is the most common gross finding
E. Staged on the pattern of pathological progression of tau protein

✅ **Answer B**

- Headache is a persistent and early symptom in nearly half the individuals who develop chronic traumatic encephalopathy. There is a long latent period (mean 8 years) between the trauma and symptoms development. Definitive diagnosis can only be made at postmortem neuropathological examination.

❓ **9. TBI-Systemic Complications**
The *FALSE* answer is:
A. Hypertension must be treated immediately and aggressively
B. Fever raises ICP

C. Incidence of venous thromboembolism up to 60% without early prophylaxis

D. Gastric ulcers progress to significant hemorrhage in up to 20%

E. Hyperglycemia associated with poor neurological outcome

✅ **Answer A**

▬ Quick reductions of hypertension in patients with untreated mass lesions are risky because CPP is maintained by this high value. Aggressive therapies could lead to cerebral hypoperfusion.

❓ **10. TBI-Headache**

The *FALSE* answer is:

A. The most common somatic complaint after TBI

B. Onset within the first day after TBI

C. Not correlated with the severity of injury

D. Estimated prevalence around 60%

E. Migraine-like is the most common type

✅ **Answer B**

▬ The International Classification of Headache Disorders defines acute and chronic posttraumatic headaches; both require the symptoms to start within 7 days and continue for more than 2 and 3 months, respectively.

❓ **11. TBI-Infections**

The *FALSE* answer is:

A. Prophylactic antibiotics: no level I evidence.

B. Early tracheostomy reduces rate of nosocomial pneumonia: no evidence

C. Povidone oral care: recommended to reduce ventilator-associated pneumonia

D. EVD antibiotics-impregnated catheters: decreases catheter-related infections

E. Periprocedural antibiotics for intubation: no mortality benefit

✅ **Answer C**

▬ The use of povidone–iodine (PI) oral care is not recommended to reduce ventilator-associated pneumonia and may cause an increased risk of acute respiratory distress syndrome.

3

❓ 12. TBI-Infections

The *FALSE* answer is:
A. Severe TBI patients are more prone to infections compared to other ICU patients.
B. Ventilator-acquired pneumonia is the most common cause within the first week.
C. Urinary catheters are common source of infection.
D. Sepsis is a major mortality contributor in severe TBI.
E. Nosocomial infections in severe TBI have no impact on neurodegeneration.

✅ Answer E

— Nosocomial infections may be the major contributors to mortality and deleterious long-term consequences as they exacerbate neurodegeneration, with neuronal loss likely impending the extent of neurological recovery.

❓ 13. TBI-Immune System

The *FALSE* answer is:
A. Secondary injury lasts up to 1 month.
B. Inflammatory mediators promote neural regeneration.
C. Microglia cells are the primary responders.
D. Impaired cell-mediated immunity increases infection risk.
E. Immune deficiency syndromes are common.

✅ Answer A

— Secondary injury involves the initiation of neuroinflammation, excitotoxicity, oxidate stress, necrosis, and apoptosis, which may last for weeks to years.

❓ 14. TBI-Hydrocephalus

The *FALSE* answer is:
A. Ventriculomegaly is symptomatic in one-third of patients
B. Traumatic SAH is not a validated risk factor
C. Severity of brain injury is the most important risk factor
D. Late decompressive craniectomy (DC) increases the risk
E. Associated with worse outcomes

✔️ **Answer D**

– Timing of decompressive craniectomy or cranioplasty is not related to hydrocephalus development. Severity of TBI is the most important risk factor.

❓ **15. TBI-Hydrocephalus.**
   The *FALSE* answer is:
   A. The most common neurosurgically treatable complication in the rehabilitation setting
   B. Time scale of symptoms is used to differentiate it from atrophic ventriculomegaly
   C. Lumbar puncture is useful diagnostic tool
   D. Correlates significantly with epilepsy development after 1 year
   E. All cases require shunting

✔️ **Answer E**

– In obstructive hydrocephalus, ventricular shunting is the definitive treatment. In communicating hydrocephalus, repeated lumbar punctures may suffice and obviate the need for a shunt. CT ventricles measurement, single photon emission computed tomography (SPECT), lumbar puncture and MRI aqueduct flow measurement are useful diagnostic tools.

❓ **16. TBI-Outcome Predictors**
   The *FALSE* answer is:
   A. Age
   B. EEG findings
   C. Pupils
   D. GCS score
   E. Brain CT findings

✔️ **Answer B**

– EEG has not been shown to reliably predict outcome following severe TBI except in the case of absent EEG activity, in which case it indicates brain death in the normotensive, normothermic patient.

❓ **17. TBI-Hypopituitarism**
   The *FALSE* answer is:
   A. Pituitary stalk necrosis is the most common postmortem finding.
   B. Incidence of hypopituitarism is 27%.
   C. Growth hormone is the most commonly affected.

3

D. Low GCS is a risk factor for hypopituitarism.
E. Ischemic insult is the cause of hypopituitarism.

✅ **Answer A**
- Postmortem findings in patients with posttraumatic hypopituitarism include capsular hemorrhage around the pituitary (59%), posterior lobe hemorrhage (31%), anterior lobe necrosis (22%), and stalk necrosis (3%).

❓ **18. TBI-Major Depressive Disorder (MMD)**
The *FALSE* answer is:
A. Prevalence is low
B. Present with mild TBI
C. Dorsolateral frontal and temporal lesions found in most of the patients
D. More severe post-concussive symptoms
E. SSRIs first line

✅ **Answer A**
- Major depressive disorder is the most prevalent psychiatric disorder after TBI, with a prevalence of up to 42% and 61%, during the first and next seven years following the insult, respectively.

❓ **19. TBI-Cardiovascular Complications**
The *FALSE* answer is:
A. Hypertension
B. Hypotension
C. No raised cardiac biomarkers
D. Pulmonary edema
E. Arrhythmias

✅ **Answer C**
- The spectrum of cardiovascular complications includes blood pressure fluctuations, ECG changes, arrhythmias, autonomic instability, cardiac injury biomarkers, left ventricular dysfunction, and pulmonary edema.

❓ **20. Depressed Fractures**
The *FALSE* answer is:
A. Compound: high risk of seizures
B. All bone fragments forced inward breaching the dura must be elevated

C. Antibiotics are needed in some cases
D. Closed: repair for cosmesis
E. Compound: close observation in normal GCS

✅ **Answer B**
- If a compound depressed fracture overlies the posterior two-thirds of the superior sagittal sinus or transverse sinus, elevation of the fragments may lead to a profuse bleeding. It is prudent to perform a wound toilet avoiding removal of fragments where the risks outweigh the potential benefits. Compound depressed fractures have high risk of seizures, infections, and mortality.

❓ **21. Glasgow Outcome Score (GOS)**
The *FALSE* answer is:
A. GOS 0: Death
B. GOS 2: Neurovegitative
C. GOS 3: Severe disability
D. GOS 4: Moderate disability
E. GOS 5: Good recovery

✅ **Answer A**
- No GOS of 0 exists. GOS of 1 = death.

❓ **22. Outcome: RESCUEicp Trial**
The *FALSE* answer is:
A. ICP >25 mmHg for 1–12 h randomized to either barbiturates or DC.
B. Unilateral hemicraniectomy or bifrontal decompressive craniectomy (DC) was performed.
C. DC was found to have higher mortality than medical management.
D. DC group had higher rate of vegetative state.
E. Moderate disability and good recovery were similar in both groups.

✅ **Answer C**
- RESCUEicp (Trial of Decompressive Craniectomy for Traumatic Intracranial Hypertension) compares decompressive craniectomy to medical management for refractory increased ICP after TBI.
- Conclusions: decompressive craniectomy in patients with TBI and refractory intracranial hypertension resulted in lower mortality and higher rates of vegetative state, lower severe disability, and upper severe disability than medical care.

3

❓ 23. Outcome DECRA Trial

The *FALSE* answer is:

A. Craniectomy group had a lower functional outcome than standard care group.
B. DC was effective in decreasing the ICP.
C. DC was associated with higher ICU time.
D. One of the limitations is that clinicians were aware of study-group assignments.
E. ICP >20 mmHg for 15 minutes within 1 hour period was the treatment threshold.

✅ Answer C

— The DECRA trial/2011 (Decompressive Craniectomy in Patients with Severe Traumatic Brain Injury) attempted to determine the value of decompressive craniectomy in patients with diffuse, severe TBI with high intracranial pressures. Bifrontal decompressive craniectomy, compared with standard care, decreased the mean intracranial pressure and the duration of both ventilatory support and the ICU stay but was associated with a significantly worse Extended Glasgow Outcome Scale at 6 months.

❓ 24. Outcome: Pupillometry

The *FALSE* answer is:

A. Pupillary responsiveness is useful to predict neurological impairment.
B. The mean constriction velocity decreases when ICP is above 20 mmHg.
C. Accuracy of pupillometer measurements is equal to the naked eye assessment.
D. Neurological pupil index (NPi) <3 is considered abnormal.
E. Propofol and barbiturates may decrease the constriction velocity thus alter the NPi.

✅ Answer C

— Quantitative pupillometry provides reliable measurements with a low error rate compared to the naked eye pupillary assessment, allowing to predict neurological impairment due to life-threatening transtentorial herniation up to 7.4 h in advance.

❓ 25. TBI: Prognosis Indicators
The *FALSE* answer is:
A. Apolipoprotein E alleles: poor
B. Age over 65: poor
C. Penetrating: high early mortality rate
D. Severe TBI: cognitive impairment
E. Repeated minor concussions: no prognostic evidence

✅ Answer E
- Athletes involved in contact sports who have sustained minor concussion have been studied. There is evidence that three or more concussions are associated with cumulative effects and increased risk for future concussions.

Suggested Reading

Carney N, Totten AM, O'Reilly C, Ullman JS, Hawryluk GW, Bell MJ, Bratton SL, Chesnut R, Harris OA, Kissoon N, Rubiano AM. Guidelines for the management of severe traumatic brain injury. Neurosurgery. 2017;80(1):6–15.
Jones KE, Puccio AM, Harshman KJ, Falcione B, Benedict N, Jankowitz BT, Stippler M, Fischer M, Sauber-Schatz EK, Fabio A, Darby JM. Levetiracetam versus phenytoin for seizure prophylaxis in severe traumatic brain injury. Neurosurg Focus. 2008;25(4):E3.
Oh JW, Kim SH, Whang K. Traumatic cerebrospinal fluid leak: diagnosis and management. Korean J Neurotrauma. 2017;13(2):63.
Prosser JD, Vender JR, Solares CA. Traumatic cerebrospinal fluid leaks. Otolaryngol Clin N Am. 2011;44(4):857–73.
Phang SY, Whitehouse K, Lee L, Khalil H, McArdle P, Whitfield PC. Management of CSF leak in base of skull fractures in adults. Br J Neurosurg. 2016;30(6):596–604.
Donald PJ. Neurosurgery: skull base craniofacial trauma. J Neurolog Surg Part B, Skull base. 2016;77(5):412.
Ott L, Young B, Phillips R, McClain C, Adams L, Dempsey R, Tibbs P, Ryo UY. Altered gastric emptying in the head-injured patient: relationship to feeding intolerance. J Neurosurg. 1991;74(5):738–42.
Daneshvar DH, Goldstein LE, Kiernan PT, Stein TD, McKee AC. Post-traumatic neurodegeneration and chronic traumatic encephalopathy. Mol Cell Neurosci. 2015;66:81–90.
Wijayatilake DS, Sherren PB, Jigajinni SV. Systemic complications of traumatic brain injury. Curr Opin Anaesthesiol. 2015;28(5):525–31.
Hoffman JM, Lucas S, Dikmen S, Braden CA, Brown AW, Brunner R, Diaz-Arrastia R, Walker WC, Watanabe TK, Bell KR. Natural history of headache after traumatic brain injury. J Neurotrauma. 2011;28(9):1719–25.
Farrell D, Bendo AA. Perioperative management of severe traumatic brain injury: what is new? Curr Anesthesiol Rep. 2018;8(3):279–89.

3

Kourbeti IS, Vakis AF, Papadakis JA, Karabetsos DA, Bertsias G, Filippou M, Ioannou A, Neophytou C, Anastasaki M, Samonis G. Infections in traumatic brain injury patients. Clin Microbiol Infect. 2012;18(4):359–64.

Smrcka M, Mrlian A, Klabusay M. Immune system status in the patients after severe brain injury. Bratisl Lek Listy. 2005;106(3):144–6.

Sharma R, Garg K. Role of decompressive Craniectomy in traumatic brain injury—how much wiser are we after randomized evaluation of surgery with craniectomy for uncontrollable elevation of intracranial pressure trial? Neurosurgery. 2017;81(5):E58–60.

Honeybul S, Ho KM. Incidence and risk factors for post-traumatic hydrocephalus following decompressive craniectomy for intractable intracranial hypertension and evacuation of mass lesions. J Neurotrauma. 2012;29(10):1872–8. Guidelines of hydo mx following tbi

Haveman ME, Van Putten MJ, Hom HW, Eertman-Meyer CJ, Beishuizen A, Tjepkema-Cloostermans MC. Predicting outcome in patients with moderate to severe traumatic brain injury using electroencephalography. Crit Care. 2019;23(1):1–9.

Tan CL, Hutchinson PJ. A neurosurgical approach to traumatic brain injury and post-traumatic hypopituitarism. Pituitary. 2019;22(3):332–7.

Fann JR, Hart T, Schomer KG. Treatment for depression after traumatic brain injury: a systematic review. J Neurotrauma. 2009;26(12):2383–402.

Gregory T, Smith M. Cardiovascular complications of brain injury. Contin Educ Anaesth Crit Care Pain. 2012;12(2):67–71.

Ahmad S, Afzal A, Lal Rehman FJ. Impact of depressed skull fracture surgery on outcome of head injury patients. Pak J Med Sci. 2018;34(1):130.

Shukla D, Devi BI, Agrawal A. Outcome measures for traumatic brain injury. Clin Neurol Neurosurg. 2011;113(6):435–41.

Hutchinson PJ, Kolias AG, Timofeev IS, Corteen EA, Czosnyka M, Timothy J, Anderson I, Bulters DO, Belli A, Eynon CA, Wadley J. Trial of decompressive craniectomy for traumatic intracranial hypertension. N Engl J Med. 2016;375:1119–30.

Cooper DJ, Rosenfeld JV, Murray L, Arabi YM, Davies AR, D'Urso P, Kossmann T, Ponsford J, Seppelt I, Reilly P, Wolfe R. Decompressive craniectomy in diffuse traumatic brain injury. N Engl J Med. 2011;364(16):1493–502.

Bower MM, Sweidan AJ, Xu JC, Stern-Nezer S, Yu W, Groysman LI. Quantitative pupillometry in the intensive care unit. J Intensive Care Med. 2019;10:0885066619881124.

Tasaki O, Shiozaki T, Hamasaki T, Kajino K, Nakae H, Tanaka H, Shimazu T, Sugimoto H. Prognostic indicators and outcome prediction model for severe traumatic brain injury. J Trauma Acute Care Surg. 2009;66(2):304–8.

Spinal Neurotrauma

Contents

Chapter 4   Principles and Initial Assessment – 65

Chapter 5   Management of Spinal Neurotrauma – 95

Chapter 6   Complications, Outcomes, and Other Aspects – 121

Principles and Initial Assessment

*Ameya S. Kamat, Ali A. Dolachee,
Mohammed A. Al-Dhahir, Abdullah H. Al Ramadan,
Mohammed A. Al-Rawi, Fatima O. Ahmed,
Zahraa F. Al-Sharshahi, and Samer S. Hoz*

Contents

Suggested Reading – 91

© The Author(s), under exclusive license to Springer Nature Switzerland AG 2022
S. S. Hoz et al., *Neurotrauma*, https://doi.org/10.1007/978-3-030-80869-3_4

4

? 1. Subaxial spine trauma: pathophysiology
The *FALSE* answer is:
A. Subaxial spine provides is responsible of the majority of forward and lateral flexion of the neck
B. Subaxial spine provides 50% of cervical rotation
C. In adults, 75% of cervical injuries occur in the subaxial region
D. Children are more prone to subaxial than occipito-cervical injuries
E. Holdsworth two-column theory is used to assess the stability

✓ Answer D
- Children are more prone to occipito-cervical injuries than subaxial ones, due to their ligamentous laxity, incompletely ossified vertebral bodies, and underdeveloped neck muscles, all of which predispose them to occipito-cervical injuries.

? 2. Subaxial spine trauma: mechanism of injury
The *FALSE* answer is:
A. Hyperflexion is the most common type of injury
B. C5–C6 is the most frequently injured level
C. Wedge fracture results from hyperflexion
D. Tear drop fracture results from severe hyperflexion and axial loading
E. Clay-shoveler fracture results from hyperflexion injury only

✓ Answer E
- While clay-shoveler fracture is usually caused by sudden neck flexion, it can also occur by direct blow to the spinous process of C7 or by whiplash injury.

? 3. Subaxial spine trauma: fracture types
The *FALSE* answer is:
A. Wedge fracture is always considered stable
B. Tear-drop fracture is usually considered unstable
C. Unlike flexion tear-drop fractures, extension tear-drop fractures are stable
D. Subluxation maybe associated with bony fractures or dislocations
E. Unilateral facet dislocation is more stable than the bilateral one

✓ Answer A
- Wedge fracture with more than 50% loss of vertebral height and/or compression fracture with significant retropulsed bony fragment,

should be considered unstable due to the higher likelihood of an associated ligamentous injury.

4. Hyperextension subaxial cervical spine injuries
The *FALSE* answer is:
A. More common in the young
B. Most damage the anterior longitudinal ligament
C. Result in fractures in posterior column bony elements
D. Most are considered stable
E. Usually results in cord impaction

Answer A
– In subaxial cervical spine, the hyperextension injuries are most likely to occur in the elderly due to underlying cervical spondylosis.

5. Whiplash injuries
The *FALSE* answer is:
A. Symptoms always start immediately
B. Traumatic injury to soft tissue structures in the region of the cervical spine
C. Due to hyperflexion, hyperextension, or rotational injury
D. Complaints include headaches, cognitive impairment, and low back pain
E. Most common nonfatal automobile injury

Answer A
– Symptoms usually develop gradually.

6. Whiplash injuries
The *FALSE* answer is:
A. Results from contact injury to the neck
B. Implies propulsive force to the head and neck complex
C. Neck sprain
D. Soft tissue neck injury
E. Usually conservatively managed

Answer A
– The whiplash injury results from acceleration force, as rear-end impact to occupants in a stationary vehicle, which should be distinguished from the contact injury, where direct impact to the neck results in a spectrum of fractures and dislocations.

? 7. Clay-shoveler's fracture

The *FALSE* answer is

A. Traumatic avulsion of the spinous process
B. Most commonly affects C7
C. A stable fracture and usually possess no risk
D. Strenuous contraction of the trapezius and rhomboid muscles
E. Not associated with whiplash injuries

4

✓ Answer E

▬ Frequently associated with whiplash injuries and other injuries that jerk the arms upward. May also occur due to direct contact with the spinous process.

? 8. Soft collars

The *FALSE* answer is

A. No significant impact on preventing lateral rotation
B. May be indicated in minor cervical spine trauma
C. Reminds the patient to reduce neck movements
D. May be difficult to apply in patients with severe kyphotic deformities
E. Prevents flexion at mid-cervical levels

✓ Answer E

▬ Soft collars have no significant impact on preventing lateral rotation. It is imporatnt to remind the patient their injury so that they reduce neck movements.

? 9. Cervical traction

The *FALSE* answer is

A. The pin in Gardener Wells tongs must be inserted into the outer table of the skull only
B. There should be no crushing of the skin
C. Reduction traction requires up to one-third of the patient's body weight
D. Presence of skull fractures is an absolute contraindication to the application of cranial tongs
E. The correct weights to apply equate to 2.5 Kg for the head and 0.5 Kg for every level up to the injured level

✓ Answer D

━ Not all skull fractures prohibit the application of cranial tongs; yet, a meticulous understanding of the fracture lines is required if tongs are to be placed. A skull fracture is a contraindication when the fracture pattern could result in depressed skull fracture or an extension of the original fracture due to proximity of cranial tongs placement. Patients must be able to obey commands so that their neurology can be frequently assessed when applying cervical traction.

❓ 10. Occipital condyle fractures

The *FALSE* answer is:

A. Occipito-cervical fusion is recommended in bilateral fractures with gross instability
B. Halo immobilization is commonly used in the management of unilateral fractures
C. Cervical collars are often used in the management of stable undisplaced fractures
D. MRI is recommended to assess ligamental integrity as ligaments are often compromised
E. AP cervical spine X-ray is the investigation of choice

✓ Answer E

━ CT and MRI are both required. CT assesses the fracture and degree of displacement. MRI assesses ligamental integrity. AP and lateral cervical spine X-ray views often are inefficient due to superimposition of nearby structures (i.e., maxilla, occiput, mastoid processes).

❓ 11. Type II odontoid fractures, factors associated with non-union

The *FALSE* answer is

A. Displacement > 6 mm
B. Angulation = 5 degrees
C. Inadequate immobilization
D. Large surface area at the fracture site
E. TAL interposition

✓ Answer B

━ Angulation of 10 degrees or more is associated with an increased risk of nonunion.

4

? 12. "Jumped facets"

The _FALSE_ answer is:

A. Results from flexion/distraction of the cervical spine
B. The inferior facets of the upper vertebra become locked in the intervertebral foramena
C. The inferior articular process is completely anterior to the articular surface of the superior articular process of the inferior vertebra
D. Approximately 10% of bilateral facet dislocations result in quadriplegia
E. Direct axial loading is a common cause

✓ Answer D

━ Bilateral facet dislocation of the cervical spine results in complete spinal cord lesions and quadriplegia in 50–84% of the cases.

? 13. Cervical fractures/dislocations

The _FALSE_ answer is

A. Atlantoaxial instability is secondary to injury to the apical ligament
B. The cervical spine is the most frequently injured portion of the spinal column
C. The axis is the most frequently injured level, followed by C5 and C6
D. Jefferson fractures are burst fractures of the atlas.
E. Posterior arch of C1 fractures result from a compression–hyperextension injury

✓ Answer A

━ Atlantoaxial instability is secondary to injury to the transverse ligament. This can be a purely ligamentous injury or may involve an avulsion fracture of the tubercle.

? 14. Spinal cord injury without radiographic abnormality (SCIWORA)

The _FALSE_ answer is:

A. Commonest in teenagers
B. Increased risk in patients with asymptomatic Chiari I malformation
C. Attributed to increased elasticity of the spinous ligaments and paravertebral soft tissue in younger populations

D. Surgical intervention, namely, laminectomy, has shown minimal benefit in recovery
E. Rigid cervical collar has a role in management

✅ **Answer A**
- Commonest in children aged below the age of 10 due to increased ligamental laxity.

❓ **15. Hangmans fracture**
The *FALSE* answer is:
A. Traumatic fracture dislocation of C2/3
B. Type I is unstable and needs surgical fixation
C. Type II must be reduced and treated in a halo vest
D. Type III is unstable and all require either anterior C2–C3 or posterior C1–C3 fusion
E. Most commonly due to falls in the elderly

✅ **Answer B**
- Type I usually treated with external orthosis for three months.

❓ **16. Initial evaluation and management of spinal trauma**
The *FALSE* answer is:
A. Spinal immobilization is essential in suspected trauma
B. Systolic blood pressure must be maintained at >90 mmHg
C. Nasogastric tubes are contraindicated
D. Indwelling catheters must be inserted to prevent urinary retention
E. Hypovolemia must be avoided

✅ **Answer C**
- Nasogastric (NG) tubes are contraindicated in the base of skull fracture. In spine trauma, NG tubes are indicated to prevent vomiting and aspiration and to decompress the abdomen which can interfere with respirations if distended (paralytic ileus is common and may last several days).

❓ **17. Epidemiology of spinal cord injury (SCI)**
The *FALSE* answer is:
A. Up to 90% of cases are traumatic
B. Younger patients have worse outcomes

C. Bimodal age distribution: young adults and patients over 60 years
D. Males are more commonly affected in adulthood and women in adolescence
E. Male-to-female ratio is 2:1

✓ Answer B
- Adults older than 60 years of age who suffer SCI have considerably worse outcomes than younger patients, and their injuries usually result from falls and age-related bony changes

4

? 18. Frankel Grading in SCI
The *FALSE* answer is:
A. Grade A—complete loss of sensory and motor function below the level of injury
B. Grade B—complete motor loss with preserved sensory function
C. Grade C—incomplete motor loss without practical use.
D. Grade D—some motor preservation, motor grade = 2
E. Grade E—normal sensory and motor function

✓ Answer D
- The Frankel Grading System in SCI was developed in 1969. It is a functional classification. Frankel D represents some useful motor function which can be graded >3/5.

? 19. American Spinal Injury Association (ASIA) Scoring System
The *FALSE* answer is:
A. Grade A—Complete loss of motor function only, below the level of injury
B. Grade B—Sensation is preserved below the level of injury
C. Grade C—Motor function below the level of injury is preserved, with more than half of the main muscles receiving a less than 3 grade on the ASIA motor score
D. Grade D—Motor function below the level of injury is preserved, with more than half of the main muscles receiving at least a 3 or greater grade on the ASIA motor score
E. Grade E—Normal sensation and motor function

✅ **Answer A**
- Complete loss of motor and sensory function below the level of injury
- Developed in 1984 by the America Spinal Cord Injury Association
- The validity and reproducibility of ASIA system combined with its accuracy in predicting patients' outcome have made it the most accepted and reliable clinical scoring system utilized for neurological classification of SCI

❓ **20. Central Cord Syndrome (CCS)**

The *FALSE* answer is:
A. Commonest incomplete SCI syndrome
B. Occurs in 15–25% of traumatic SCI
C. Commoner in elderly patients
D. Due to decreased blood supply to watershed regions in the central part of the spinal cord
E. CCS is characterized by disproportionately greater motor impairment in lower compared to upper extremities

✅ **Answer E**
- In CCS, the upper limb weakness is disproportionately greater than that of the lower limbs. Other neurologic manifestations include sensory impairment and bladder dysfunction.

❓ **21. Anterior Cord Syndrome (ACS)**

The *FALSE* answer is
A. Occlusion of the anterior spinal artery
B. Above C7 may result in quadriplegia
C. Damage to the anterior one-third of the spinal cord with sparing of the posterior two-thirds
D. Affects spinothalamic tract—loss of pain and temperature sensation
E. Worst prognosis of incomplete SCI syndromes

✅ **Answer C**
- Results from damage to the anterior two-thirds of the spinal cord with sparing of the posterior one-third. Posterior columns not affected hence there is preservation of two-point discrimination, proprioception, and deep pressure sensation. Only ≈10–20% recover functional motor capacity.

? 22. Acute traumatic central cord syndrome (ATCCS)

The *FALSE* answer is:

A. The upper extremities are weaker than the lower with variable sensory system and bladder function
B. It constitutes 70% of the acute incomplete spinal cord injuries
C. 10% have MRI signal changes within the cord with no other radiographic changes
D. Less than 5% present with acute disc herniation
E. 30% of ATCCS cases have cervical spine skeletal injuries

✓ Answer D

━ Almost 20% of ATCCS patients have acute disc herniation.
━ Surgical intervention is recommended in these cases.

? 23. Posterior cord syndrome

The *FALSE* answer is:

A. Known as contusio cervicalis posterior
B. Relatively rare form of incomplete SCI syndromes
C. Pain and paresthesia in the upper limbs and torso
D. Minimal long tract signs
E. Best prognosis among incomplete SCI syndromes

✓ Answer E

━ Brown–Sequard syndrome is the incomplete spinal cord injury with the best prognosis, as 90% of patients will regain independent ambulation, along with the sphincters control.
━ Posterior cord syndrome (contusio cervicalis posterior) is relatively rare and causes bilateral loss of vibration and proprioception below the level of the lesion. If the injury was large enough, it may disrupt the corticospinal tracts resulting in mild paresis.

? 24. Spinal examination

The *FALSE* answer is:

A. C5 dermatome—deltoid area
B. C7 dermatome—dorsal aspect of little finger
C. T1 dermatome—medial aspect of forearm
D. L4 dermatome—medial malleolus
E. S1 dermatome—lateral aspect of foot

✓ **Answer B**

- The C7 dermatome is best examined by palpating the skin over the dorsum of the middle finger. The dorsal aspect of the little finger is represented by the C8 dermatome.

? **25. Spinal examination**

The *FALSE* answer is:

A. L5 myotome—extensor hallucis longus
B. C7 myotome—elbow extension (triceps)
C. C5 myotome—arm abduction (deltoid)
D. L4 myotome—ankle plantar flexion
E. C8 myotome—finger flexors

✓ **Answer D**

- L4 myotome is involved in inversion and ankle dorsiflexion.

Myotomes	
C1, C2	Cervical flexion
C3	Cervical side flexion
C4	Scapula elevation
C5	Shoulder abduction
C6	Elbow flexion and wrist extension
C7	Elbow extension and wrist flexion
C8	Thumb extension
T1	Finger abduction
L1, L2	Hip flexion
L3	Knee extension
L4	Ankle dorsiflexion
L5	Big toe extension
S1	Ankle plantiflexion
S2	Knee flexion

❓ 26. Spinal examination

The *FALSE* answer is:

A. Bicep reflex—C5/6
B. Brachioradialis reflex—C6
C. Triceps reflex—C7/8
D. Knee reflex—L1/L2
E. Ankle reflex—S1/2

4

✅ Answer D

- The L3 and L4 myotomes are responsible for the knee reflex.

Deep tendon reflex	Muscle involved	Nerve supply	Root supply
Biceps	Biceps	Musculocutaneous	C5, C6
Triceps	Triceps	Radial	C6, C7, C8
Pectoralis	Pectoralis major	Pectoral	C6, C7, C8
Brachioradialis	Brachioradialis	Radial	C5, C6
Finger flexors	Flexor digitorum	Median and ulnar	C7, C8, T1
Knee	Qadriceps femoris	Femoral	L2, L3, L4
Adductor	Adductors	Obturator	L2, L3, L4
Ankle	Soleus/gastrocnemius	Sciatic/tibial	S1, S2
Plantar	Small foot muscle	Plantar	S1

❓ 27. Radiographic signs of cervical trauma

The *FALSE* answer is:

A. Loss of lordosis
B. Atlantodental interval (ADI) >3 mm in children
C. Widening of apophyseal joints
D. Tracheal deviation
E. Acute kyphotic angulation

✅ Answer B

- The atlantodental interval is a measure of the distance between the posterior aspect of the anterior arch of C1 and the anterior aspect of the dens. Normal measurements in adults are under 3 mm and up to 5 mm in children.

❓ 28. Spinal shock

The *FALSE* answer is:

A. Loss of sensation accompanied by motor paralysis with initial loss but gradual recovery of reflexes following SCI
B. Different than neurogenic shock which is due to lack of sympathetic outflow after SCI
C. Circulatory collapse
D. Reflexes return in 1–3 days post injury
E. Hyperreflexia occurs after the first week

✅ Answer C

— Although termed spinal shock, there is no circulatory collapse which occurs in hypovolemic, neurogenic, and septic shock.

❓ 29. Spinal shock.

The *FALSE* answer is

A. Phase 1 – Areflexia or hyporeflexia
B. Phase 2 – Initial reflex return
C. Phase 3 – Hyperreflexia (initial)
D. Phase 4 – Hyperreflexia (late)
E. Phase 5 – Spasticity

✅ Answer E

— There are only 4 described phases in spinal shock. Spasticity occurs in phase four.

❓ 30. Jefferson classification of C1 fractures.

The *FALSE* answer is

A. Type I – single arch fracture
B. Type I – usually avulsion fractures with low morbidity
C. Type II – caused by direct axial loading
D. Type III – fracture of lateral mass
E. Type IV – burst fracture

✅ Answer C

— Type II – caused by hyperextension

> **◻ Table 4.1**   Traynelis Classification
>
> Type I – anterior subluxation (commonest)
>
> Type II – vertical distraction
>
> Type III – posterior dislocation (rarest)

4

❓ 31. Atlanto-occipital dissociation.
   The *FALSE* answer is
   A. Rupture of alar ligaments, tectorial membrane, and occipito-atlantal joint capsules
   B. May cause subarachnoid hemorrhage at the craniocervical junction
   C. Flexion and distraction or rotation and hyperextension
   D. 10% mortality rate
   E. Anderson and D'Alonzo classification is used to classify atlanto-occipital dissociation (AOD)

✅ Answer E
   ▬ Classified by the Traynelis classification (◻ Table 4.1):

❓ 32. Odontoid fractures.
   The *FALSE* answer is
   A. Represent 15% of C2 fractures
   B. Bimodal age distribution
   C. Neurological deficits in 10–20% of cases
   D. Hyperflexion injury mechanism is common.
   E. Type II fractures have the highest risk of non-union

✅ Answer A
   ▬ Odontoid fractures represent 60% of C2 fractures (the most common C2 fracture) and 10–15% of all cervical spine fractures.
   ▬ Classified by Anderson and D'Alonzo classification
   ▬ Due to low-energy falls in the elderly and high-energy mechanisms in the young

■ **Table 4.2**   Indications for surgery in penetrating spine Injuries

Incomplete lesions
CSF leak
Nerve root compression
Retained copper jacket bullet
Worsening neurological deficit
Infection prevention (military gun shot wound (GSW's))

❓ 33. Indications for surgery in penetrating spine injuries.

The *FALSE* answer is

A. CSF leak
B. Complete lesions
C. Vascular injuries
D. Instability
E. Neurologic deterioration

✅ Answer B

- Indications for surgery are shown in ■ Table 4.2:

❓ 34. Denis' Three Column theory in thoracolumbar fractures.

The *FALSE* answer is

A. Anterior column: anterior half of disc and vertebral body + anterior longitudinal ligament
B. Compression fractures usually involve the anterior column only
C. Middle column: posterior half of disc and vertebral body+ posterior longitudinal ligament
D. Posterior column: posterior bony complex + posterior ligamentous complex
E. Burst fractures affect the middle and posterior columns

✅ Answer E

- Burst fractures are axial loading injuries. They involve the anterior and middle columns. Usually occur between T10 and L2.
- The posterior ligamentous complex: supraspinous and interspinous ligament, facet joints and capsule, and ligamentum flavum.

35. Burst fractures of the thoracolumbar spine.

The *FALSE* answer is

A. 50% are neurologically intact at initial examination
B. 5% have complete paraplegia
C. Anterior and middle columns involved
D. Hyperextension injury
E. Occur mainly at the thoracolumbar junction

Answer D
- Burst fractures occur due to direct axial loading + flexion
- The posterior column is spared
- Inferior endplate involvement is rare

36. Brown Sequard-syndrome (BSS).

The *FALSE* answer is

A. Poor prognosis
B. Hemisection of the spinal cord
C. Affects the corticospinal tract, dorsal columns and spinothalamic tract
D. Contralateral loss of pain and temperature sensation
E. May result in Horners syndrome if the lesion is above T1

Answer A
- BSS is an incomplete spinal cord injury due to hemisection of the cord. It is characterized by spastic paralysis and loss of deep pressure and vibration sensation on the same side as the injury and contralateral loss of pain and temperature sensation. It has the best prognosis among the incomplete spinal cord syndromes.

37. Traumatic spinal epidural hematoma (SEH).

The *FALSE* answer is

A. 0.5% to 1.7% of all spinal injuries
B. Ankylosing spondylitis is a risk factor
C. 16% of cases involve the cervical spine
D. The thoracic spine involved in the young and lumbar spine in the elderly
E. MRI is the gold standard investigation

Answer D
- Young patients usually suffer from SEH in the lumbar spine. The elderly usually sustain SEH in the thoracic spine. Spontaneous SEH occur in patients with AVM, intramedullary tumours, and hemophilia.

- Risk factos include ankylosing spondylitis, rheumatoid arthritis, arteriorvenous malformations, and spinal tumours.
- MRI is superior to CT, as opposed to cranial EDH.

38. Clinical clues to spine injury in a comatose patient
The *FALSE* answer is
A. Bradycardia with hypotension
B. Priapism
C. Horner syndrome
D. Dissociation of core and surface body temperatures
E. Hypertonicity of the limbs

Answer E
- Most severe brain injuries cause hypertonicity but flaccid Paralysis is an alerting sign to the presence of a spinal cord injury in a comatose patient.
- Bradycardia with hypotension may indicate neurogenic shock (disruption of autonomic pathways)

39. MRI in spinal trauma.
The *FALSE* answer is:
A. Short tau inversion recovery (STIR) sequence evaluates edema.
B. Better visualization of paravertebral soft tissues.
C. Alignment and vertebral marrow signal can be evaluated through T1-weighted sagittal sections.
D. T1 sequence is preferred over T2 sequence.
E. Cerebrospinal fluid is "bright" in T2 Sequences.

Answer D
- T2 weighted sequences can better evaluate vertebral height, pars interarticularis, longitudinal, interspinous, and supraspinous ligaments, central spinal canal, epidural space, spinal cord, disk contour, pedicles, spinal cord, lateral recess, neural foramina, facet joints, epidural space, curvature of spine, paravertebral soft tissues, and sacroiliac joints. The T2 sequence is therefore is preferred over T1 weighted MRI sequences.

40. Normal cervical spine biomechanics
The *FALSE* answer is:
A. 20 to 40 degrees of lordosis
B. Frontal plane: 35 degrees of lateral flexion.
C. Sagittal plane: flex up to 65 degrees.

D. Sagittal plane: extend up to 55 degrees.
E. Normal axial rotation with respect to the sagittal plane is approximately 50 degrees bilaterally

✅ **Answer D**
- In the sagittal plane, the cervical spine can normally extend up to 40 degrees.

4

❓ **41. AOSPINE thoracolumbar spinal injury classification.**
The *FALSE* answer is:
A. Type A3: incomplete burst fracture
B. Type C: translation/displacement
C. NX: complete cord injury
D. M1: can help identify unstable fractures due to ligamentous injury
E. Multilevel injuries are classified individually and listed in order of severity.

✅ **Answer C**
- NX: patient cannot be examined
- The AOSpine classification asseses three major components: (1) fracture morphology, (2) neurologic status, and (3) patient-specific modifiers and comorbidities (◻ Table 4.3).

◻ **Table 4.3**   AOSPINE Thoracolumbar Spine Injury Classification

1. Fracture Morphology	2. Neurologic Status	3. Clinical Modifiers

A: compression
  A0: minor injuries
  A1: wedge compression
  A2: split/pincer
  A3: incomplete burst
  A4: complete burst
B: tension band
  B1: monosegment bony tension band
  B2: posterior tension band with type A
  B3: hyperextension
C: translation/displacement
	N0: Intact
	N1: Transient deficit
	N2: Radiculopathy
	N3: Incomplete cord/cauda equina
	N4: Complete cord
	NX: Unable to examine
		M1: Fractures with an indeterminate injury to the PLC or posterior tension band on either clinical examination or imaging studies.
		M2: patient-specific comorbidity that may either call for or hinder potential surgical intervention.

- MI: can help identify unstable fractures seem stable from a bony standpoint but have a ligamentous component that may render them unstable.

42. Post-traumatic blood-spinal cord barrier (BSCB) distrubtion.
The *FALSE* answer is:
A. A malfunctioning BSCB has decreased permeability.
B. Occurs as a consequence of the primary impact of trauma.
C. Secondary proinflammatory mediators are implicated.
D. Results in cranio-caudal expansion of the primary injury lesion.
E. Induces spinal oedema.

Answer A
- Malfunction of the affected BSCB leads to an increase in its permeability.

43. Occipital-cervical junction
The *FALSE* answer is:
A. Responsible for 13 to 21 degrees of flexion and extension of the cervical spine.
B. Limited in rotation and lateral bending.
C. Occipital-C1 junction injuries: compression and distraction.
D. Dislocation injuries occur more often in adults than in children
E. No occipital-atlanto disc exists.

Answer D
- Atlanto-occipital dislocations are encountered more often in children than in adults due to: (1) more ligamentous laxity in children (2) relatively large head and high fulcrum
- The occipital-cervical junction is limited in rotation and lateral bending, with only 7 degrees of rotation and 5 degrees of lateral bending.

? **44. Quebec Task force grading of Whiplash-Associated Disorder (WAD),**
The *FALSE* answer is:
A. Grade 0: no neck complaints and no physical sign of injury
B. Grade 1: neck pain, tenderness, and stiffness
C. Grade 2: decreased range of motion and point tenderness
D. Grade 3: arm heaviness, fatigue, and paresthesias
E. Grade 4: cervical fractures and/or dislocations

4

✓ **Answer A**
- Unlike Gargan and Bannister whiplash-associated disorder (WAD) classification, Quebec Task Force grading of Whiplash-Associated Disorder does not have a grade 0.

? **45. Traumatic spinal cord edema.**
The *FALSE* answer is:
A. Abnormal local venous circulation
B. May be misinterpreted as an inflammatory condition.
C. hyperintense on T2W imaging and isointense of T1W imaging
D. Lower proportion of gadolinium enhancement than patients with cervical spondylotic myelopathy
E. Spinal decompression is the mainstay in acutely deteriorating patients

✓ **Answer D**
- Patients with cervical spondylotic myelopathy (CSM) rarely have gadolinium enhancement of the spinal cord.

? **46. Standalone external orthoses in spinal trauma.**
The *FALSE* answer is
A. Type I Hangman's fractures
B. Post-operative control of spine fractures
C. Anterior vertebral body fractures
D. Type IIa Hangman's fracture
E. Stable cervical spine fractures

✓ **Answer D**
- Unstable cervical spine fractures require surgical stabilization or external orthoses such as a halo vest. An orthosis may be used in the post-operative phase to allow for healing. Type IIa Hangman fractures are highly unstable and require surgical stabilization.

❓ 47. Seatbelt injuries.
  The *FALSE* answer is
  A. May result in intestinal injuries
  B. Compression injury of the anterior spinal column
  C. Occur as a result of the interaction between the restrained occupant and the belt
  D. Distraction injury of the middle and posterior spinal columns
  E. A missing seat belt injury implies that the belt was not used

✅ Answer E
  ▬ Seat belt injures typically occur following frontal motor vehicle collisions. The absence seat belt sign may imply that the belt might have been rolled out because of pre-crash movements of the occupant, or the impact was not purely frontal.
  ▬ The typical seat belt sign – a skin abrasion running diagonally across the chest (shoulder belt) and/or across the lower abdomen (lap belt)

❓ 48. Pre-hospital spine immobilization.
  The *FALSE* answer is:
  A. Firm application of a cervical collar associated with increased ICP
  B. Pressure ulcer development depends on time spent on rigid board
  C. Routinely used in penetrating trauma
  D. Cervical injury associated with other spinal injury in 20% of cases.
  E. Up to 25% of spinal cord injuries occur after initial insult

✅ Answer C
  ▬ Penetrating trauma (stab and gunshot) rarely causes spinal instability. Cervical collar immobilization leads to unrecognized penetrating injury and delays patient resuscitation hence its routine use is not recommended.

❓ 49. Pre-hospital spinal immobilization criteria.
  The *FALSE* answer is:
  A. Significant multi-system injuries
  B. Any neck pain with a history of trauma
  C. Severe head or facial trauma

4

D. Criteria are 99% sensitive with cervical injuries requiring immobilization,
E. Both soft and hard collar can be used

✅ **Answer E**
- Cervical immobilization must be hard collar
- Pre-hospital spinal immobilization is advised when there is: (i) spinal pain or tenderness, including any neck pain with a history of trauma, (ii) significant multiple system trauma, (iii) severe head or facial trauma, (iv) numbness or weakness in any extremity after trauma, (v) loss of consciousness caused by trauma, (vi) mental status is altered (including drugs, alcohol, trauma) (vii) any significant injury distracting the patient from reporting spinal pain/symptoms. These criteria are 99% sensitive in identifying trauma patients with cervical injuries requiring immobilization.

❓ **50. Cervical bracing.**
The *FALSE* answer is:
A. Soft collar used to immobilize the neck
B. Rigid collar is inadequate for immobilizing the upper and midcervical spine
C. Poster brace good for preventing flexion of midcervical spine
D. Halo-vest immobilizes upper and lower C-spine
E. Halo-vest may cause snaking of midcervical levels

✅ **Answer A**
- Soft collar dose not significantly immobilize the cervical spine. It's used mostly to remind the patient to reduce neck movements.

❓ **51. Radiological image indication in cervical trauma according to the NEXUS study.**
The *FALSE* answer is:
A. Sensitivity of 99.6% for ruling out cervical spine injury
B. Midline spinal tenderness
C. Patient >65 years of age
D. Focal neurologic deficit
E. Distracting injury

✅ **Answer C**
- The NEXUS = National Emergency X-ray Utilization Study criteria used to define trauma patients who do not require imaging:
  1. Alert and stable
  2. No focal neurological deficit
  3. No alter level of consciousness
  4. Not intoxicated no midline tenderness
  5. No distracting injury
- Nexus is not a reliable tool for patient more than 65 years

❓ **52. Canadian C-spine rules in cervical injury imaging.**
The *FALSE* answer is:
  A. ≥65 years
  B. Fall from >3 feet
  C. Paresthesia in extremities
  D. Low-risk injury: no further imaging.
  E. High-speed motor vehicle collision

✅ **Answer D**
- If the patient meets the criteria for a low-risk injury, then one should assess whether the patient can rotate the neck 45°
- if low-risk injury and the patient can rotate the neck 45°, no cervical spine imaging required
- if low-risk injury and the patient cannot rotate the neck 45°, then cervical spine imaging is warranted

❓ **53. Bulbocavernous (BC) reflex.**
The *FALSE* answer is:
  A. Polysynaptic reflex
  B. Mediated via S2-4 nerve roots
  C. Can be lost in spinal shock
  D. Can be lost in injuries to conus or cauda equine
  E. Its return is the last sign of spinal shock recovery

✅ **Answer E**
- Return of the BC reflex is the earliest clinical indicator that spinal shock has subsided, but its presence alone is not longer an indicator of a good prognosis for recovery.

4

② 54. Flexion injuries of the thoraco-lumbar spine.
The *FALSE* answer is:
A. Distruption of the middle & posterior columns.
B. Flexion of the spine along an axis anterior to the anterior column
C. "Chance" fractures can be easily detected by CT-scan
D. "Chance" fractures are associated with abdominal injuries without neurological deficits
E. Usually managed surgically with posterior instrumental fusion

✔ Answer C
- Chance fractures are unstable horizontal fractures that are associated with abdominal organs injuries in 50% of the cases, but can be easily missed by CT scans if the fracture happens to fall between axial cuts.

② 55. Subaxial Cervical Spine Injury Classification and Severity Scale (SLIC)
The *FALSE* answer:
A. Score 2: Discoligamentous complex disruption
B. Score 3: Incomplete cord injury
C. Score 2: Complete cord injury
D. Score 3: Burst fracture
E. Score 4: Unstable teardrop fracture

✔ Answer D
- Burst fractures are SLIC score 2
- Subaxial injury classification and severity score system SLIC (◘ Table 4.4)

◘ **Table 4.4** SLIC Scoring System

Morphology		Discoligamentous complex		Neurological status	
Characteristic	Point	Characteristic	Point	Characteristic	Point
No abnormality	0	Intact	0	Intact	0
Compression	1	Intermediate	1	Root injury	1
Burst	2	Disrupted	2	Complete SCI	2
Distraction	3			Incomplete SCI	3
Rotation / translation	4			Continuous cord compression	+1

? **56. Punjabi and White stability of mid and lower cervical criteria.**
The *FALSE* answer is:
A. Cord or root damage: 2 points
B. Relative sagittal plane rotation >11° on X-ray: 2 points
C. Relative sagittal plane translation >3.5 mm on X-ray: 2 points
D. Posterior elements destroyed or unable to function: 2 points
E. A total of 5 points or more suggests spinal instability

✔ **Answer A**
– White and Panjabi guidelines for diagnosing clinical instability of the mid & lower C-spine

Item	Points
Anterior elements destroyed	2
Posterior elements destroyed	2
Positive stretch test	2
Spinal cord damage	2
Nerve root damage	1
Abnormal disc narrowing	1
Narrow spinal canal, either sagittal diameter < 13 mm, OR Pavlov ratio < 0.8	1
Dangerous loading anticipated	1

? **57. Spinal cord injury without radiographic abnormality (SCIWORA)**
The *FALSE* answer is:
A. Common in the pediatric population
B. Signs and symptoms of cord injury
C. Described before the MRI era
D. MRI is always unremarkable
E. Related to ligamentous laxity

✔ **Answer D**
– MRI may show evidence of discoligamentous disruption and spinal cord injury

4

? **58. Spinal cord injury without radiological abnormality.**

The *FALSE* answer is:

A. Normal MRI scan in 35%

B. Responsible for 9–14% of spinal injuries in adults.

C. Conservative management is the mainstay approach.

D. The use of high dose steroids lacks level-1 evidence.

E. Bracing is maintained for 1 month during which only noncontact sports are allowed.

✓ Answer E

— Bracing is maintained for 3 months, during which both contact and noncontact sports are strictly prohibited

? **59. Anderson and Montesano classification for occipital condyle fractures**

The *FALSE* answer is:

A. Type I is the least common

B. Type I is comminuted, results from axial loading

C. Type II is an extension of base of skull fracture

D. Type III is an avulsion fracture

E. Type III portends worst outcome

✓ Answer A

— Type I is the most commonly recognized type on high resolution CT-scan

Anderson & Montesano classification of occipital condyle fractures		
Type	Description	Management
I	Comminuted from impact: may occur from axial loading	+/− external immobilization (collar or halo)
II	Extension of linear basilar skull fracture	
III	Avulsion of condyle fragment	external immobilization (collar or halo)

Suggested Reading

1. Aarabi B, Walters BC, Dhall SS, et al. Subaxial cervical spine injury classification systems. Neurosurgery. 2013;72(Suppl 2):170–86.
2. Wang TY, Mehta VA, Dalton T, Sankey EW, Goodwin CR, Karikari IO, Shaffrey CI, Than KD, Abd-El-Barr MM. Biomechanics, evaluation, and management of subaxial cervical spine injuries: a comprehensive review of the literature. J Clin Neurosci. 2020;83:131.
3. Feuchtbaum E, Buchowski J, Zebala L. Subaxial cervical spine trauma. Curr Rev Musculoskelet Med. 2016;9(4):496–504.
4. Zaveri G, Das G. Management of sub-axial cervical spine injuries. Indian J Orthop. 2017;51:633–52.
5. Radanov BP, Sturzenegger M, Di Stefano G. Long-term outcome after whiplash injury. A 2-year follow-up considering features of injury mechanism and somatic, radiologic, and psychosocial findings. Medicine. 1995;74(5):281–97.
6. Geiger G, Aliyev RM. Whiplash injury as a function of the accident mechanism. Neuro-otological differential diagnostic findings. Unfallchirurg. 2012;115(7):629–34.
7. Olivier EC, Muller E, van Rensburg DC. Clay-shoveler fracture in a paddler: a case report. Clin J Sport Med. 2016;26(3):e69–70.
8. Barati K, Arazpour M, Vameghi R, Abdoli A, Farmani F. The effect of soft and rigid cervical collars on head and neck immobilization in healthy subjects. Asian Spine J. 2017;11(3):390.
9. Morin M, Langevin P, Fait P. Cervical spine involvement in mild traumatic brain injury: a review. J Sports Med. 2016;2016:1590161.
10. Hadley MN, Walters BC, Grabb PA, Oyesiku NM, Przybylski GJ, Resnick DK, Ryken TC. Occipital Condyle Fractures. Neurosurgery. 2002;50(suppl_3):S114.
11. Guan J, Bisson EF. Treatment of odontoid fractures in the aging population. Neurosurg Clin N Am. 2017;28(1):115–23.
12. Anissipour AK, Agel J, Baron M, Magnusson E, Bellabarba C, Bransford RJ. Traumatic cervical unilateral and bilateral facet dislocations treated with anterior cervical discectomy and fusion has a low failure rate. Global Spine J. 2017;7(2):110–5.
13. Siddiqui J, Grover PJ, Makalanda HL, Campion T, Bull J, Adams A. The spectrum of traumatic injuries at the craniocervical junction: a review of imaging findings and management. Emerg Radiol. 2017;24(4):377–85.
14. Li X-F, Dai L-Y, Lu H, Chen X-D. A systematic review of the management of hangman's fractures. Eur Spine J. 2005;15(3):257–69. https://doi.org/10.1007/s00586-005-0918-2.
15. Ghiselli G, Schaadt G, McAllister DR. On-the-field evaluation of an athlete with a head or neck injury. Clin Sports Med. 2003;22:445–65.
16. Kang Y, Ding H, Zhou H, Wei Z, Liu L, Pan D, Feng S. Epidemiology of worldwide spinal cord injury: a literature review. J Neurorestoratol. 2017;6:1–9.
17. Frankel HL, Hancock DO, Hyslop G, Melzak J, Michaelis LS, Ungar GH, et al. The value of postural reduction in the initial management of closed injuries of the spine with paraplegia and tetraplegia. Paraplegia I. 1969;7:179–92. https://doi.org/10.1038/sc.1969.30.
18. American Spinal Injury Association. International standards for neurological classification of spinal cord injury, revised 2000. 6th ed. Chicago: American Spinal Injury Association; 2000.

19. Penrod LE, Hegde SK, Ditunno JF. Age effect on prognosis for functional recovery in acute, traumatic central cord syndrome. Arch Phys Med Rehabil. 1990;71:963–8.
20. Foo D, Rossier AB. Anterior spinal artery syndrome and its natural history. Paraplegia. 1983;21(1):1–10.
21. Aarabi B, Hadley MN, Dhall SS, Gelb DE, Hurlbert RJ, Rozzelle CJ, Ryken TC, Theodore N, Walters BC. Management of acute traumatic central cord syndrome (ATCCS). Neurosurgery. 2013;72(Suppl 2):195–204.
22. McKinley W, Hills A, Sima A. Posterior cord syndrome: demographics and rehabilitation outcomes. J Spinal Cord Med. 2021;44(2):241–6.
23. McKinley W, Santos K, Meade M, Brooke K. Incidence and outcomes of spinal cord injury clinical syndromes. J Spinal Cord Med. 2007;30(3):215–24.
24. Downs MB, Laporte C. Conflicting dermatome maps: educational and clinical implications. J Orthop Sports Phys Ther. 2011;41(6):427–34.
25. Stifani N. Motor neurons and the generation of spinal motor neuron diversity. Front Cell Neurosci. 2014;8:293. https://doi.org/10.3389/fncel.2014.00293.
26. Dick JP. The deep tendon and the abdominal reflexes. J Neurol Neurosurg Psychiatry. 2003;74(2):150–3.
27. Clark WM, Gehweiler JA, Laib R. Twelve significant signs of cervical spine trauma. Skelet Radiol. 1979;3:201–5.
28. Hakova R, Kriz J. Spinal shock-from pathophysiology to clinical manifestation. CESKA A SLOVENSKA NEUROLOGIE A NEUROCHIRURGIE. 2015;78(3):263–7.
29. Ditunno JF, Little JW, Tessler A, Burns AS. Spinal shock revisited: a four-phase model. Spinal Cord. 2004;42(7):383–95.
30. Jefferson G. Fractures of the atlas vertebra: report of four cases, and a review of those previously recorded. Br J Surg. 1920;7:407–22.
31. Theodore N, Aarabi B, Dhall SS, Gelb DE, Hurlbert RJ, Rozzelle CJ, Ryken TC, Walters BC, Hadley MN. The diagnosis and management of traumatic atlanto-occipital dislocation injuries. Neurosurgery. 2013;72(Suppl 2):114–26.
32. Gonschorek O, Vordemvenne T, Blattert T, Katscher S, Schnake KJ. Spine Section of the German Society for Orthopaedics and Trauma. Treatment of odontoid fractures: recommendations of the spine section of the German Society for orthopaedics and trauma (DGOU). Global Spine J. 2018;8(2_suppl):12S–7S.
33. Kumar A, Pandey PN, Ghani A, Jaiswal G. Penetrating spinal injuries and their management. J Craniovertebral Junction Spine. 2011;2(2):57.
34. Denis F. The three column spine and its significance in the classification of acute thoracolumbar spinalinjuries. Spine. 1983;8:817–31.
35. Heary RF, Kumar S. Decision-making in burst fractures of the thoracolumbar and lumbar spine. Indian J Orthopaed. 2007;41(4):268.
36. Ranga U, Aiyappan S. Brown-Séquard syndrome. Indian J Med Res. 2014;140(4):572–3.
37. Egido Herrero JA, Saldanã C, Jiménez A, Vázquez A, Varela de Seijas E, Mata P. Spontaneous cervical epidural hematoma with Brown-Séquard syndrome and spontaneous resolution. Case report. J Neurosurg Sci. 1992;36(2):117–9.
38. Tian HL, Guo Y, Hu J, Rong BY, Wang G, Gao WW, Chen SW, Chen H. Clinical characterization of comatose patients with cervical spine injury and traumatic brain injury. J Trauma Acute Care Surg. 2009;67(6):1305–10.

39. Kumar Y, Hayashi D. Role of magnetic resonance imaging in acute spinal trauma: a pictorial review. BMC Musculoskelet Disord. 2016;17(1):1–1.

40. Bogduk N, Mercer S. Biomechanics of the cervical spine. I: Normal kinematics. Clin Biomech. 2000;15(9):633–48.

41. Vaccaro AR, Oner C, Kepler CK, Dvorak M, Schnake K, Bellabarba C, Reinhold M, Aarabi B, Kandziora F, Chapman J, Shanmuganathan R. AOSpine thoracolumbar spine injury classification system: fracture description, neurological status, and key modifiers. Spine. 2013;38(23):2028–37.

42. Jin LY, Li J, Wang KF, Xia WW, Zhu ZQ, Wang CR, Li XF, Liu HY. Blood–spinal cord barrier in spinal cord injury: a review. J Neurotrauma. 2021;38:1203.

43. Offiah CE, Day E. The craniocervical junction: embryology, anatomy, biomechanics and imaging in blunt trauma. Insights Imaging. 2017;8(1):29–47.

44. Pastakia K, Kumar S. Acute whiplash associated disorders (WAD). Open Access Emerg Med. 2011;3:29–32.

45. Magu S, Singh D, Yadav RK, Bala M. Evaluation of traumatic spine by magnetic resonance imaging and correlation with neurological recovery. Asian Spine Jl. 2015;9(5):748.

46. Johnson RM, Hart DL, Simmons EF, et al. Cervical orthoses. A study company their effectiveness in restricting cervical motion in normal subjects. J Bone Joint Surg Am. 1977;59:332–9.

47. Eberhardt CS, Zand T, Ceroni D, Wildhaber BE, La Scala G. The seatbelt syndrome-do we have a chance?: a report of 3 cases with review of literature. Pediatr Emerg Care. 2016;32(5):318–22. https://doi.org/10.1097/PEC.0000000000000527. PMID 26087444

48. Theodore N, et al. Prehospital cervical spinal immobilization after trauma. Neurosurgery. 2013;72(Suppl 3):22–34.

49. Dixon M, O'Halloran J, Cummins NM. Biomechanical analysis of spinal immobilization during prehospital extrication: a proof of concept study. Emerg Med Journal: EMJ. 2014;31(9):745–9.

50. Horodyski M, DiPaola CP, Conrad BP, Rechtine GR II. Cervical collars are insufficient for immobilizing an unstable cervical spine injury. J Emerg Med. 2011;41(5):513–9.

51. Paykin G, O'Reilly G, Ackland H, Mitra B. NEXUS criteria to rule out cervical spine injury among older patients: a systematic review. Emerg Med Australas. 2018;30(4): 450–5.

52. Canadian C-spine rule and the National Emergency X-Radiography Utilization Study (NEXUS) for detecting clinically important cervical spine injury following blunt trauma. Cochrane Database Syst Rev. 2018;(4):Art. No.: CD012989.

53. Ko HY. Revisit spinal shock: pattern of reflex evolution during spinal shock. Korean J Neurotrauma. 2018;14(2):47.

54. Desai J. Beevors sign. Ann Indian Acad Neurol. 2012;15(2):94.

55. Grossbach AJ, Dahdaleh NS, Abel TJ, Woods GD, Dlouhy BJ, Hitchon PW. Flexion-distraction injuries of the thoracolumbar spine: open fusion versus percutaneous pedicle screw fixation. Neurosurg Focus. 2013;35(2):E2.

56. Joaquim AF, Patel AA, Vaccaro AR. Cervical injuries scored according to the subaxial injury classification system: an analysis of the literature. J Craniovertebral Junction Spine. 2014;5(2):65.

57. White III AA, Panjabi MM. Clinical biomechanics of the spine.

4

58. Atesok K, Tanaka N, Robinson Y, Pittman J, Theiss S. Current best practices and emerging approaches in the management of acute spinal trauma.
59. Szwedowski D, Walecki J. Spinal cord injury without radiographic abnormality (SCIWORA)–clinical and radiological aspects. Pol J Radiol. 2014;79:461.
60. Rozzelle CJ, Aarabi B, Dhall SS, et al. Spinal cord injury without radiographic abnormality (SCIWORA). Neurosurgery. 2013;72(Suppl 2):227–33.
61. Anderson PA, Montesano PX. Morphology and treatment of occipital condyle fractures. Spine. 1988;13:731–6.
62. Traynelis VC, Marano GD, Dunker RO, Kaufman HH. Traumatic atlanto-occipital dislocation. Case report. J Neurosurg. 1986;65:863–70.
63. Vaccaro AR, Hulbert RJ, Patel AA, Fisher C, Dvorak M, Lehman RA, Jr, et al. The subaxial cervical spine injury classification system: A novel approach to recognize the importance of morphology, neurology, and integrity of the disco-ligamentous complex. Spine (Phila Pa 1976) 2007;32:2365–74.

Management of Spinal Neurotrauma

Redab A. Alkhataybeh, Hazem Madi,
Baha'eddin A. Muhsen, Ali A. Dolachee,
Mohammed A. Al-Dhahir,
and Zahraa F. Al-Sharshahi

Contents

Suggested Reading – 117

? 1. **Methylprednisolone for treatment of acute spinal cord injury (SCI).**
The *FALSE* answer is:
A. There is no class II evidence supporting benefit in the treatment of acute SCI.
B. Class I evidence suggesting harmful effects of high dose of steroids on all body systems.
C. No evidence to support the neuroprotective effect of methylprednisolone in acute SCI.
D. The accepted dose is 30 mg/kg bolus then 5.4 mg/kg/h. for the next 24 h (if <3-h post-injury).
E. Maintenance of mean arterial pressure (MAP) 80–90 mmHg for the first 7 days is safe and improves cord perfusion and outcome.

✅ **Answer C**
- A variety of class III medical evidence (NASCIS) has been published supporting the neuroprotective effect of methylprednisolone in SCI, but these studies suffer from limitations like sample size and incomplete data reporting.

? 2. **Traumatic atlanto-occipital dislocation (AOD).**
The *FALSE* answer is:
A. More common in pediatrics.
B. Hyper-flexion injury mechanisms.
C. 20% have normal neurological examination on presentation.
D. Pre-vertebral soft tissue swelling on lateral c-spine prompt CT imaging.
E. Power's ratio >1 suggests AOD.

✅ **Answer B**
- AOD results from hyperextension and distraction of the cervical spine, resulting in disruption of the craniocervical junction, due to ligamentous injuries.
- Found in 8–19% of fatal cervical spine injury autopsies.
- Power's ratio (Basion-Posterior atlas distance divided by Opsthion-Anterior atlas distance) >1 is a radiographic parameter suggesting AOD.

? 3. **Traumatic AOD, management**
The *FALSE* answer is:
A. Accounts for <1% of all acute cervical spine injuries.

B. Dublin measure is 60% sensitive.
C. Basion-axial interval (BAI) >12 mm in adults.
D. Atlanto-occipital interval (AOI) >2 mm in adults.
E. All symptomatic patients should be treated with craniocervical fixation.

✅ **Answer B**
- Dublin measure is one of the methods used in radiographic evaluation of AOD. It is 25% sensitive. Normally, the mandible to anterior atlas ratio is ≤13 mm and mandible to dens ≤20 mm.

❓ 4. **Traumatic AOD, radiographic evaluation.**
The *FALSE* answer is:
A. BAI is better for type I and type III AOD.
B. Basion-dental interval (BDI) is better for type II AOD.
C. Normal BAI and BDI in adults ≤12 mm on plain radiographs.
D. BAI should never be negative in pediatrics.
E. Normal AOI ≤2 mm in pediatrics.

✅ **Answer E**
- AOD is classified into three types according to the relative dislocation of the occiput to the atlas. Type I is anterior dislocation, type II is distracted dislocation, and type III is posterior dislocation. While the normal AOI (condylar gap) is ≤2 mm in adults, the normal pediatric value is ≤5 mm.

❓ 5. **Closed reduction of cervical spine fracture-dislocation injuries.**
The *FALSE* answer is:
A. MRI must be done before any attempted reduction in all patients.
B. MRI is recommended for patients who fail closed reduction.
C. MRI will demonstrate disrupted intervertebral discs.
D. Early closed reduction restores anatomic alignment of the cervical spine.
E. Muscle relaxants may help facilitate reduction.

✅ **Answer A**
- Patients with cervical spine fracture-dislocation injuries who are not conscious and cannot be examined during attempted closed reduction should undergo MRI study before the attempted reduction.

 — Muscle relaxant or analgesic, such as diazepam or meperidine, may help facilitate reduction.

? 6. **Closed reduction of cervical fracture-dislocations.**
    The *FALSE* answer is:
    A. Risk of transient injury is 2–4%.
    B. Risk of permanent neurological injury is 1%.
    C. Weight increments used in Gardener Wells tongs is 15 lb per level.
    D. The more rostral the dislocation, the less weight is used in the longitudinal traction.
    E. Contraindicated when power's ratio >1.

✓ **Answer C**
 — This technique involves use of longitudinal traction using skull tongs or a halo headpiece. An initial weight of 5–15 pounds is applied; this is increased in 5 lb increments, taking lateral X-rays after each increment is applied. The more rostral the dislocation, the less weight is used, usually about 3–5 pounds per vertebral level. While weights up to 70 pounds are sometimes used, it is suggested that after 35 pounds is applied, patients be observed for at least an hour with repeat cervical spine X-rays before the weight is cautiously increased further.

? 7. **Occipital condyle fractures.**
    The *FALSE* answer is:
    A. Cervical collars are the mainstay of treatment.
    B. MRI is recommended to assess the integrity of craniocervical ligaments.
    C. Cervical collars are contraindicated in the presence of cranial nerve palsy.
    D. Type III: avulsion of a fragment.
    E. Type II: extension of a linear basilar skull fracture.

✓ **Answer C**
 — Nonsurgical treatment with external cervical immobilization is sufficient to promote bony union/healing and recovery or cranial nerve deficit improvement in nearly all types of occipital condyle fractures (OCF). Yet it is worthy to know that fusion might be indicated in rare cases where instability is present (■ Table 5.1).

◘ Table 5.1 Classification of occipital condyle fractures

Anderson and Montesano classification		Tuli et al. classification	
Type I	Nondisplaced comminuted fracture. Axial loading-*stable fracture*	Type I	Non-displaced fracture – may not require stablization
Type II	Fracture through skull base extending to condyle. *stable fracture*	Type II	(displaced fracture)
Type III	Avulsion fracture of ipsilateral condyle by alar ligament. Unstable fracture	IIA	No ligamentous instability, may require external stabilization
		IIB	Ligamentous instability, may require surgical fixation

❓ 8. Atlas (C1) fracture.
   The *FALSE* answer is:
   A. Comprises 2–13% of all cervical fractures.
   B. 50% incidence of associated cervical fractures.
   C. Results in poor outcome.
   D. Jefferson type results from symmetrical axial load.
   E. Stability is defined by the integrity of the transverse ligament.

✔ Answer C
   ▬ Atlas fractures often have good outcomes, as the fractured components of the ring tend to expand away from the cord.

❓ 9. Odontoid fractures.
   The *FALSE* answer is:
   A. Hyperextension or hyperflexion injury.
   B. Classified by Anderson and D'Alonzo into three types.
   C. Type I is the least common and generally stable.
   D. Type II has the most predictable healing rate.
   E. Type III is stable with better union rates.

✔ Answer D
   ▬ Type II has unpredictable healing and high risk of non-union, especially in elderly >50 years old with translation >6 mm, failed reduction, or angulation >10° (◘ Table 5.2).

5

⬛ **Table 5.2**   Anderson and D'Alonzo classification of odontoid fractures

Type I	An oblique fracture line through the upper part of the odontoid process representing an avulsion fracture
Type II	A fracture at the junction between the odontoid process and the body of the axis
Type IIA	Similar to type II but with fragments of bone present at the fracture site
Type III	A fracture that extends down into the cancellous bone of the body of the axis and, in reality, is a fracture of the body of C2

❓ **10. Indications for surgery in odontoid fractures.**
   The *FALSE* answer is:
   A. Age >7years and <50 years.
   B. Instability of the fracture on halo vest.
   C. Displacement >5 mm.
   D. Disruption of the transverse ligament.
   E. Hadley Type IIa fractures.

✅ **Answer A**
— Elderly, >50-year-old are at high risk of nonunion (21-fold) with external immobilization, and surgical intervention should be considered.

❓ **11. Os odontoideum.**
   The *FALSE* answer is:
   A. Anatomic variant of the odontoid process of C2.
   B. May represent an old nonunion fracture.
   C. Trauma is the only cause.
   D. Asymptomatic patients treated conservatively.
   E. C1–2 instabilities treated by posterior C1–2 internal fixation and fusion.

✅ **Answer C**
Os odontoideum etiology
1. Congenital: developmental anomaly (nonunion of dens to body of the axis).
2. Acquired: postulated to represent an old nonunion fracture.

❓ **12. Hangman fracture.**
   The *FALSE* answer is:
   A. Bilateral fractures of the isthmus of C2.

B. Comprises 15% of cervical fractures.
C. Civilian hangman fractures result from hyperflexion with axial loading.
D. 95% of patients are neurologically intact.
E. Surgical management is not always indicated.

✅ **Answer C**
— Most modern civilian hangman fracture (HF) result from hyperextension and axial loading which differs from that sustained in judicial hangings (hyperextension and distraction). Some cases may be due to forced flexion or compression of the neck while in extension.

❓ **13. Hangman fracture types.**
The *FALSE* answer is:
A. Type I has no angulation, <3 mm translation.
B. Type II has disruption of posterior longitudinal ligament (PLL) and C2-3 disc.
C. Type IIa has less displacement and more angulation.
D. Type III has disrupted anterior longitudinal ligament (ALL) and C2-C3 facet capsules.
E. All should be managed with reduction and halo vest.

✅ **Answer E**
— Type I is stable managed with collar only. Type III is highly unstable and should be managed by open surgical reduction of dislocated facets with C1-2 or C1-3 lateral mass fusion.

❓ **14. Treatment of subaxial cervical spine fractures**
The *FALSE* answer is:
A. Management is based on the total SLIC score.
B. Anterior immobilization and fusion indicated in most flexion injuries.
C. Posterior immobilization and fusion indicated in most extension injuries.
D. Anterior approach indicated in fractured vertebral body with bone retropulsed into spinal canal.
E. Posterior immobilization and fusion indicated in unilateral or bilateral locked facets.

✅ **Answer B**
— Posterior immobilization and fusion is indicated in most flexion injuries.

? 15. Thoracolumbar fractures.
The *FALSE* answer is:
A. Burst fracture is the most common.
B. Classified by the three-column model of Denis.
C. Wedge fracture involves only anterior column.
D. Fracture dislocation may involve all three columns.
E. Seat-belt involves middle and posterior columns.

✓ Answer A
— Wedge fracture is the most common in thoracolumbar fracture. They are usually stable and managed conservatively.

5

? 16. Unstable thoracolumbar compression fractures
The *FALSE* answer is
A. Single compression fracture with loss of >50% of height with angulation.
B. Excessive kyphotic angulation at one segment >15°.
C. Progressive kyphosis when >75% loss of height.
D. Three or more contiguous compression fractures.
E. Spinal cord or nerve root injury.

✓ Answer B
Unstable compression fractures
1. A single compression fracture with:
   (a) Loss of >50% of height with angulation (particularly if the anterior part of the wedge comes to a point).
   (b) Excessive kyphotic angulation at one segment (various criteria are used, none are absolute. Values quoted: >30°, >40°).
2. Three or more contiguous compression fractures.
3. Neurologic deficit (generally does not occur with pure compression fracture).
4. Disrupted posterior column or more than minimal middle column failure.
5. Progressive kyphosis: risk of progressive kyphosis is increased when loss of height of anterior vertebral body is >75%. Risk is higher for lumbar compression fractures than thoracic.

? 17. Thoracolumbar burst fractures.
The *FALSE* answer is:
A. Failure of both anterior and middle columns.

B. >50% loss of vertebral body height.
C. >20° segmental kyphosis.
D. 20% have neurological deficits.
E. Generally treated with surgical decompression and fixation.

✅ **Answer D**
 ▬ Almost 50% of patients with thoracolumbar burst fractures have neurological deficits.

❓ **18. Thoracolumbar injury classification and severity score (TLICS).**
The *FALSE* answer is:
A. Integrity of posterior ligamentous complex disrupted: score 3.
B. Distraction fracture: score 4.
C. Nerve root injury: score 1.
D. Cauda equina syndrome: score 3.
E. Surgical candidates if the sum score is 5 or more.

✅ **Answer C**
 ▬ According to the TLICS, the presence of a nerve root injury gives a score of 2 (◻ Table 5.3).

◻ **Table 5.3**   Thoracolumbar injury classification and severity score (TLICS)

Category	Finding	Points
Radiographic findings:	Compression fx	Score is 1
	Burst fracture or lateral angulation >15°	Score is 2
	Distraction fracture	Score is 4
	Translational/rotational injury	Score is 3
Posterior ligamentous complex:	Intact	0
	Undetermined	2
	Injured	3
Neurologic status:	Intact	0
	Root injury	2
	Complete SCI	2
	Incomplete SCI	3
	Cauda equine syndrome	3

❓ 19. Osteoporotic spine fractures.
The *FALSE* answer is:
A. Lifetime risk for females is 16%.
B. Increased risk with phenytoin use.
C. DEXA scan is the best test.
D. Lumbar spine bone marrow density (BMD) measurement is the best predictor for future fractures.
E. Lumbar spine is the best location to assess response to treatment.

5

✅ Answer D
Dual energy X-ray absorptiometry (DEXA) scan: the preferred way to measure BMD.
1. Proximal femur: bone marrow density (BMD) measurement in this location is the best predictor for future fractures.
2. Lumbar spine (LS): best location to assess response to treatment.

❓ 20. Osteoporotic spine fractures.
The *FALSE* answer is:
A. DEXA scan T-score: norms for healthy young adults.
B. DEXA scan Z-score: norms of subjects of same age and sex as the patient.
C. Osteoporosis: T score < – 2.5 SD.
D. Increased calcium intake is effective in preventing osteoporosis in adults.
E. Vertebral body augmentation to shorten the duration of pain and prevent progression of kyphosis.

✅ Answer D
— High calcium intake during childhood may increase peak bone mass. In adulthood, increased calcium intake (beyond daily requirement) is ineffective in preventing osteoporosis. Weight-bearing exercise in adulthood helps slow calcium loss from bones.

❓ 21. Denis classification of sacral fractures.
The *FALSE* answer is:
A. Zone 1: Fracture lateral to foramina.
B. Zone II: Fracture through foramina.
C. Zone III: Fracture medial to foramina.

D. Zone II fractures are always unstable.
E. Zone II fractures linked with highest rate of neurological deficit.

✅ **Answer D**
- Zone II fractures may be stable versus unstable. Those with shear component are highly unstable.
- Unstable fractures have increased risk of nonunion and poor functional outcome.
- Zone III fractures carry the highest rate of neurological deficits (two to three times that of Zone II fractures).

❓ **22. Sacral fractures.**
The *FALSE* answer is:
A. Identified in 90% of patients with pelvic fractures.
B. Usually caused by shear forces.
C. Sacrum below S2 is not essential to ambulation.
D. Zone II fractures with neurologic involvement may recover with or without surgical reduction.
E. Reduction of the ala may promote L5 recovery with Zone I fractures.

✅ **Answer A**
- Sacral fractures are uncommon. Identified in 17% of patients with pelvic fractures. Usually caused by shear forces. Neurologic deficits in patients with pelvic fractures may be due to associated sacral fractures.

❓ **23. Vertebral body augmentation.**
The *FALSE* answer is:
A. Food and drug administration (FDA) approved for use from C5 through L5.
B. Contraindicated in osteomyelitis.
C. Relatively contraindicated in acute burst fractures.
D. Lowest complication when used to treat osteoporotic compression fractures.
E. Used as pedicle screw salvage in spinal instrumental fusion.

✅ **Answer A**
- Transpedicular vertebral body augmentation is FDA approved for use from T5 through L5; however, it has been used off-label (primarily for tumor, e.g., multiple myeloma) from T1 through sacrum and has been described (for tumor) in the cervical spine using the anterior approach.

? 24. Vertebral body augmentation.
  The *FALSE* answer is:
  A. Transpedicular injection of polymethylmethacrylate (PMMA).
  B. FDA approved for treatment of compression fractures due to tumors.
  C. Contraindicated for asymptomatic fractures.
  D. Vertebroplasty more extravasation of cement than kyphoplasty.
  E. Vertebroplasty is better than kyphoplasty for height restoration.

5

✅ **Answer E**
  ▬ Kyphoplasty is similar to vertebroplasty except that in the first, a balloon is inserted into the compressed vertebral body (VB) through the pedicle. The balloon is inflated and then deflated and removed. Polymethylmethacrylate (PMMA) is injected into the thusly created defect. Potential benefits of this over vertebroplasty: there may be some restoration of height, and there may be less tendency for PMMA extravasation/embolization.

? 25. Missile injuries of the spine.
  The *FALSE* answer is:
  A. The third most common cause of SCI after motor vehicle accident and falls.
  B. Low velocity missile travels at <2000 feet/sec.
  C. The amount of kinetic energy contained in a missile = 1/2*mass*Velocity².
  D. Most are located in the cervical spine.
  E. Poor outcomes.

✅ **Answer D**
  ▬ Most of missile injures are located in thoracic region (54%) followed by lumbosacral (33%) and cervical (13%).

? 26. A direct high velocity missile (HVM) spinal injury.
  The *FALSE* answer is:
  A. Direct crush injury.
  B. Cavitation.
  C. Concussive wave.
  D. Intramedullary hematoma.
  E. Arterio-venous fistula.

✅ **Answer E**
- A-V fistula is not a direct/initial injury from HVM.

❓ **27. Indications for surgery in missile spine injuries.**
The *FALSE* answer is:
A. Incomplete neurological deficits.
B. Cauda equina syndrome.
C. Cervical cord injuries.
D. Contained pseudomeningoceles.
E. Worsening of neurological deficits.

✅ **Answer D**
- A contained pseudomeningocele is not an indication for surgery in missile spine injuries. The presence of an external CSF fistula is considered one of the indications for surgical management.

❓ **28. Penetrating non-missile spinal injuries.**
The *FALSE* answer is:
A. More common than missile injuries.
B. More in young males.
C. More frequent in the thoracic spine.
D. Majority caused by stabbing assault.
E. Have better outcome than missile injuries.

✅ **Answer A**
- Penetrating (non-missile) spinal injuries are rare. Few cases reported from India, but reports from South Africa account for the most of the large series published.

❓ **29. Neurological presentation of penetrating spine injuries.**
The *FALSE* answer is:
A. Brown-Sequard syndrome is the most common.
B. 20% of patients have complete spinal cord injuries.
C. 30% of patients may not have any neurological deficits.
D. Lead is associated with severe scarring.
E. Oxidation of the metallic fragments can deposit rust particles.

✅ **Answer D**
- Copper is associated with severe scarring and fibrosis, while lead and nickel excite less of a severe response.

5

⍰ 30. Surgery of penetrating spine injuries.
The *FALSE* answer is:
A. Removal of any foreign body only in operation room (O.R.)
B. Preparation for neck exploration.
C. Laminectomy, durotomy with stay sutures.
D. Insertion of lumbar subarachnoid drain for 5–10 days.
E. Spinal fixation is usually performed.

✅ Answer E
— Spinal stabilization is generally not required, since these injuries are stable.

⍰ 31. Penetrating neck trauma.
The *FALSE* answer is:
A. Venous injuries account for 18%.
B. Arterial injuries account for 12%.
C. Common carotid artery is the most involved.
D. Vertebral artery is the second most involved.
E. Outcome correlates with initial neurological presentation.

✅ Answer D
— Common carotid artery is the most usually involved artery, followed by the internal carotid artery (ICA) then external carotid artery (ECA) then the vertebral artery (VA).

⍰ 32. Classification of penetrating neck trauma.
The *FALSE* answer is:
A. Zone I: head of clavicle to the thoracic outlet.
B. Zone II: clavicle to angle of mandible.
C. Zone III: angle of mandible to base of skull.
D. Cerebral neurological deficits are related to spinal cord shock.
E. No preoperative angiography for actively bleeding patients.

✅ Answer D
— Cerebral neurological deficits are related to vascular injuries.

⍰ 33. Surgical exploration in penetrating neck injuries.
The *FALSE* answer is:
A. Wounds piercing the platysma.
B. Wounds entering the anterior triangle of neck.
C. Zone II injuries.

  D. Angiography-based exploration.
  E. 5% of the exploration will be negative.

✅ **Answer E**
  — About 40–60% of surgical exploration of penetrating wounds to the neck will be negative.

❓ **34. Surgical options in penetrating cervical vascular injuries.**
  The *FALSE* answer is:
  A. Endovascular therapy is suitable in select cases.
  B. Patients with active bleeding should be urgently operated.
  C. Carotid repair in minor or no neurological deficits.
  D. Carotid ligation in uncontrollable bleeding.
  E. Vertebral artery more often managed by direct repair.

✅ **Answer E**
  — The vertebral artery injuries are more often managed by ligation than direct repair, especially when bleeding occurs during exploration.

❓ **35. SCI: Arterial injuries.**
  The *FALSE* answer is:
  A. Overall incidence is 1–5% of blunt trauma patients.
  B. 10% of affected patients harbor a traumatic aneurysm.
  C. Blunt vertebral artery injuries are more common than cervical ICA injuries.
  D. Motor vehicle crashes are the most common cause.
  E. Vertebral artery injury due to a penetrating trauma is associated with high mortality.

✅ **Answer C**
  — Blunt cervical ICA injuries are more common than vertebral artery injuries among patients who have sustained blunt trauma.

❓ **36. SCI: Arterial injuries.**
  The *FALSE* answer is:
  A. Stretching of the artery is more likely to cause arterial dissection than direct blow.
  B. Cervical ICA is vulnerable during head hyperextension and contralateral rotation.

C. C1 to C3 fractures carry the highest risk for blunt cerebrovascular injuries.
D. The V2 segment is the most commonly affected in traumatic blunt VA injury.
E. More than one vessel injury is rarely seen.

✅ **Answer E**
— Multiple arterila injuries is encountered in approximately one third of cases stretching of the artery may produce an intimal tear, exposing subendothelial collagen, which initiates platelet aggregation and thrombus formation, with the potential for subsequent stenosis or occlusion of the vessel.

❓ **37. SCI: Arterial injuries**
The *FALSE* answer is:
A. Denever scale grade I: <25% luminal narrowing or raised intimal flap.
B. Denver scale grade II: ≥25% luminal stenosis or intraluminal thrombus.
C. Denver scale grade III: pseudoaneurysm.
D. Denver scale grade IV: occlusion.
E. Denver scale grade V: transection with extravasation.

✅ **Answer A**
— Denever scale grade I is <25% luminal narrowing. Raised intimal flap is considered grade II on Denver grading scale.
— Stroke rate in cervical carotid artery injury correlates with the grade of injury (◻ Table 5.4).

◻ **Table 5.4**   Denver criteria

Grade I	Irregularity of the wall or <25% luminal narrowing.
Grade II	Intramural thrombus or raised intimal flap or >25% luminal narrowing.
Grade III	Pseudoaneurysm.
Grade IV	Occlusion.
Grade V	Transection with extravasation.

❓ 38. Blunt internal carotid artery injury (BCI).

The *FALSE* answer is:

A. Cerebral ischemia most commonly due to thromboembolism.
B. Neck pain is the most common symptom.
C. CN VI is the most commonly affected cranial nerve.
D. May manifest weeks after the injury.
E. The pathognomonic sign of a carotid double lumen is rare.

✅ Answer C

- Hypoglossal nerve is the most common cranial nerve affected in blunt internal carotid artery injury.
- The III, IV, and VI cranial nerves can be affected if the dissection extends into cavernous segment.

❓ 39. Blunt internal carotid artery injury (BCI)

The *FALSE* answer is:

A. Aspirin is recommended for Denver grade I and II.
B. 7% of grade I injuries may progress to grade II or higher.
C. Heparin is recommended for grade III injuries.
D. Grade V injuries can be treated by endovascular occlusion.
E. One-third of patients with grade IV injuries will heal with anticoagulation alone.

✅ Answer E

- Grade III and IV lesions demonstrate a low rate of resolution with antithrombotic therapy alone.
- Only 5% of grade III lesions and no grade IV lesion heal with heparin.
- Reported indications for endovascular stent placement include the following:
  1. Failed medical management defined as a new ischemic event, progression of initial symptoms, or enlarging pseudoaneurysm.
  2. Stroke.
  3. Contraindications to anticoagulation.

❓ 40. Blunt vertebral artery injury (VAI)

The *FALSE* answer is:

A. CT angiography (CTA) is the imaging modality of choice.
B. Requires a multidisciplinary approach.

C. Cervical spine fractures are seen in almost all cases of VAI.
D. Anticoagulation therapy is recommended for documented VAI.
E. No role for endovascular therapy.

✅ **Answer E**
- Endovascular therapy is considered in patients with contraindication to anticoagulation and antiplatelet therapy

❓ 41. SCI: traumatic pseudoaneurysms.
The *FALSE* answer is:
A. The carotid system is more commonly affected
B. Ischemic stroke is more common than hemorrhagic stroke.
C. The fusiform subtype has a higher complication rate.
D. The fusiform subtype more likely to resolve with antiplatelet therapy.
E. Intraarterial thrombolysis carries lower morbidity compared to systemic thrombolysis.

✅ **Answer C**
- The saccular subtype is less common and has a greater risk of complications.
- The fusiform subtype is more common and more than half resolve with antiplatelet therapy.

❓ 42. SCI in pediatrics.
The *FALSE* answer is:
A. Not common.
B. Ligamentous injuries are infrequent.
C. C-spine is the most vulnerable segment.
D. Potential for physeal separation.
E. Higher fatality rate than adults.

✅ **Answer B**
- Ligamentous injuries are more frequent than actual fractures, due to the high ligamentous laxity, high head-body ratio, immaturity of the paraspinal muscles, and underdeveloped uncinate processes.

43. Indications for C-spine imaging in pediatrics
   The *FALSE* answer is:
   A. Unexplained hypotension.
   B. Neurological deficits.
   C. Posterior midline tenderness.
   D. Motor vehicle collision.
   E. Fall >3 feet height.

Answer E
   – Fall from >10 feet is an indication for C-spine imaging in the pediatric age group

44. Pseudospread of atlas in children.
   The *FALSE* answer is:
   A. >2 mm C1 on C2 overlap.
   B. Usually misdiagnosed with Jefferson's fracture.
   C. Typical age group: 3 months-4 years.
   D. >90% seen in the 2-year-old group.
   E. Trauma is a contributing factor.

Answer E
   – Trauma is not a contributing factor. It is probably a result of disproportionate growth of the atlas on the axis.

45. Cardiopulmonary instability.
   The *FALSE* answer is:
   A. Frequent despite the initial stable condition.
   B. Episodic and recurrent in the first 7 days.
   C. MAP target for first week is 60 mmHg.
   D. Systolic blood pressure >90 mmHg improves american spinal injury association (ASIA) scores.
   E. Hypotension induced by direct cord trauma.

Answer C
   – Maintenance of MAP between 85 and 90 mmHg for the first 7 days is safe and may improve the spinal cord perfusion and, ultimately, the neurological outcome.

? 46. Neurogenic shock.
The *FALSE* answer is:
A. Cord lesion above T6 level.
B. Loss of vasoconstrictor function.
C. Persistent tachycardia.
D. Skeletal muscle paralysis.
E. Venous blood pooling.

✓ Answer C
- In hypotensive shock, post spinal cord trauma, the interruption of the sympathetic pathway results in loss of vasoconstrictors and peripheral vasodilatation. The parasympathetic system is left unopposed resulting in bradycardia.

? 47. Spinal shock
The *FALSE* answer is:
A. Transient loss of all neurological function.
B. Flaccid paralysis and areflexia.
C. Typically persists for several months.
D. Loss of bulbocavernosus reflex.
E. Poor prognostic sign.

✓ Answer C
- Spinal shock typically persists for 1–2 weeks, but occasionally for few months.

? 48. Deep vein thrombosis (DVT).
The *FALSE* answer is:
A. Incidence ranges from 14% to 100%.
B. Incidence of fatal pulmonary embolism (PE) estimated as 5%.
C. Distal calf DVT rarely are sources of PE.
D. D-dimer test is highly sensitive and specific.
E. The majority of PE patients are asymptomatic.

✓ Answer D
- D-dimer test is highly sensitive, but it lacks specificity because D-dimers are found in other disease states, reducing the specificity of the test.
- Venography is considered the definitive test for DVT but is an invasive study.

- Venous ultrasound is cheap and noninvasive. Sensitivity is only 73% for distal clots, but 95% for the more dangerous proximal clots.

? **49. Anticoagulation.**
The *FALSE* answer is:
A. Low molecular weight heparin (LMWH) is effective for DVT prevention.
B. SCI patients should be routinely screened with doppler ultrasonography for clinically inapparent DVT during their acute-care admission.
C. Inferior vena cava (IVC) filters are not recommended as primary thromboprophylaxis
D. Pneumatic compression devices combined with LMWH have higher prevention rate.
E. DVT prophylaxis should be provided for a minimum of 8 weeks in SCI with limited mobility.

✓ **Answer B**
- SCI patients should NOT be routinely be screened with doppler ultrasonography for clinically inapparent DVT during their acute-care admission.

? **50. Indications for operative treatment of post spinal injury pyogenic vertebral osteomyelitis.**
The *FALSE* answer is:
A. Requires open biopsy.
B. Failure of nonsurgical management.
C. Need for open drainage of abscess.
D. Age above 60.
E. Neural decompression.

✓ **Answer D**
- Surgical treatment of Pyogenic vertebral osteomyelitis does not depend on age of patient.

? **51. Surgical management of vertebral osteomyelitis.**
The *FALSE* answer is
A. Simple laminectomy is the primary procedure for neural element compression.

B. Anterior or combined anterior-posterior approaches required in the majority of cases.
C. Posterior approach alone can be considered if there is disc space infection below the conus.
D. Refractory back pain after a period of nonoperative management is an indication for surgery.
E. Correction of progressive spinal deformity is an indication for surgery.

✅ Answer A
— Laminectomy alone is associated with deformity progression, instability, and neurologic deterioration; hence, it is not recommended.

❓ 52. Autonomic hyperreflexia.
The *FALSE* answer is:
A. Exaggerated autonomic response to normally innocence stimuli.
B. Sympathetic usually predominates.
C. Lesions at and below C8.
D. Rare in the first 12–16 weeks.
E. Norepinephrine release.

✅ Answer C
— Only patients with lesions above the splanchnic outflow are prone to develop autonomic hyperreflexia which is usually at or above C6.

❓ 53. Post spinal cord injury complex regional pain syndrome (CRPS).
The *FALSE* answer is:
A. Type I (reflex sympathetic dystrophy) demonstrates no definable nerve injury.
B. Type II (causalgia) demonstrates peripheral nerve lesion.
C. Pain disproportionate to inciting stimulus.
D. Hands and feet are most commonly affected.
E. No motor deficits or movements abnormalities.

✅ Answer E
— CRPS may reduce joint range of motion, and cause movement abnormalities, such as weakness, tremor, or dystonia along with the autonomic changes in the skin and temperature control.

❓ 54. Management of CRPS.
The *FALSE* answer is:
A. Regional anesthetic block.
B. Local anesthetic block.
C. Intrathecal baclofen.
D. Spinal cord stimulation.
E. Cordotomy.

✅ Answer E
- No role for cordotomy in the management of CRPS. Other possible surgical procedures include the following: Peripheral nerve stimulation, DBS, motor cortex stimulation, and TENS.

❓ 55. Prognostic factors of SCI.
The *FALSE* answer is:
A. Complete SCI has a higher mortality than incomplete SCI.
B. Stability of neurological outcome usually reached within a year of injury.
C. The most important predictor of neurological outcome is the severity of injury.
D. The level of injury is not predictive of functional outcomes.
E. The improvement for (ASIA B–D) higher than (ASIA A).

✅ Answer D
- The level of injury is a significant predictor of functional outcomes.

Suggested Reading

Alizadeh A, Dyck SM, Karimi-Abdolrezaee S. Traumatic spinal cord injury: an overview of pathophysiology, models and acute injury mechanisms. Front Neurol. 2019;10:282.
Al-Mahfoudh R, Beagrie C, Woolley E, Zakaria R, Radon M, Clark S, Pillay R, Wilby M. Management of typical and atypical Hangman's fractures. Global Spine J. 2016;6(3):248–56.
Alterman DM, Heidel RE, Daley BJ, Grandas OH, Stevens SL, Goldman MH, Freeman MB. Contemporary outcomes of vertebral artery injury. J Vasc Surg. 2013;57(3):741–6.
Anderson LD, D'Alonzo RT. Fractures of the odontoid process of the axis. J Bone Joint Surg. 1974;56A:1663–74.
Atkinson PP, Atkinson JLD. Spinal shock. Mayo Clin Proc. 1996;71:384–9.
Bhatoe HS, Singh P. Missile injuries of the spine. Neurol India. 2003;51(4):507.

Bracken MB. Steroids for acute spinal cord injury. Cochrane Database Syst Rev. 2002;1(1):CD001046.

Bydon M, Fredrickson V, De la Garza-Ramos R, Li Y, Lehman RA, Trost GR, Gokaslan ZL. Sacral fractures. Neurosurg Focus. 2014;37(1):E12.

Chen WH, Jiang LS, Dai LY. Surgical treatment of pyogenic vertebral osteomyelitis with spinal instrumentation. Eur Spine J. 2007;16(9):1307–16.

Consensus Development Conference. Prophylaxis and treatment of osteoporosis. Am J Med. 1991;90:107–10.

Demura S, Murakami H, Shirai T, Kato S, Yoshioka K, Ota T, Ishii T, Igarashi T, Tsuchiya H. Surgical treatment for pyogenic vertebral osteomyelitis using iodine-supported spinal instruments: initial case series of 14 patients. Eur J Clin Microbiol Infect Dis. 2015;34(2):261–6.

Denaro V, Longo UG, Maffulli N, Denaro L. Vertebroplasty and kyphoplasty. Clin Cases Miner Bone Metab. 2009;6(2):125.

Desouza RM, Crocker MJ, Haliasos N, Rennie A, Saxena A. Blunt traumatic vertebral artery injury: a clinical review. Eur Spine J. 2011;20(9):1405–16.

Duz B, Cansever T, Secer HI, Kahraman S, Daneyemez MK, Gonul E. Evaluation of spinal missile injuries with respect to bullet trajectory, surgical indications and timing of surgical intervention: a new guideline. Spine. 2008;33(20):E746–53.

Erickson RP. Autonomic hyperreflexia: pathophysiology and medical management. Arch Phys Med Rehabil. 1980;61:431–40.

Feuchtwanger MM. High velocity missile injuries: a review. J R Soc Med. 1982;75(12):966.

Fielding JW, Hensinger RN, Hawkins RJ. Os Odontoideum. J Bone Joint Surg. 1980;62A:376–83.

Fogelman MJ, Stewart RD. Penetrating wounds of the neck. Am J Surg. 1956;91:581–96.

Gelb DE, et al. Initial closed reduction of cervical spinal fracture-dislocation injuries. Neurosurgery. 2013;72:73–83.

Gopinathan NR, Viswanathan VK, Crawford AH. Cervical spine evaluation in pediatric trauma: a review and an update of current concepts. Indian J Orthop. 2018; 52:489–500.

Hadley MN, Walters BC, Grabb BC, Oyesiku NM, Przybylski GJ, Resnick DK, Ryken TC. Initial closed reduction of cervical spine fracture-dislocation injuries. Neurosurgery. 2002;50(3 Suppl):S44–50.

Hall GC, Kinsman MJ, Nazar RG, Hruska RT, Mansfield KJ, Boakye M, Rahme R. Atlanto-occipital dislocation. World J Orthop. 2015;6(2):236.

Hitchon PW, Jurf AA, Kernstine K, et al. Management options in thoracolumbar fractures. Contemp Neurosurg. 2000;22:1–12.

Hurlbert RJ, Hadley MN, Walters BC, et al. The acute cardiopulmonary management of patients with cervical spinal cord injuries. Neurosurgery. 2013;72(Suppl 2): 84–92.

Jenkins LN, Rezende-Neto JB. Current management of penetrating traumatic cervical vascular injuries. Curr Surg Rep. 2020;8:1–8.

Kakarla UK, Chang SW, Theodore N, et al. Atlas fractures. Neurosurgery. 2010;66:60–7.

Ko HY. Revisit spinal shock: pattern of reflex evolution during spinal shock. Korean J Neurotrauma. 2018;14(2):47.

Lee TS, Ducic Y, Gordin E, Stroman D. Management of carotid artery trauma. Craniomaxillofac Trauma Reconstr. 2014;7(3):175–89.

Levine AM. The Cervical Spine Research Society Editorial Committee. Traumatic spondylolisthesis of the axis: "Hangman's fracture". In: The cervical spine. 3rd ed. Philadelphia: Lippincott-Raven; 1998. p. 429–48.

Lo J, Cavazos J, Burnett C. Management of complex regional pain syndrome. In: Baylor University medical center proceedings, vol. 30. Taylor & Francis; 2017. p. 286–8.

Maschmann C, Jeppesen E, Rubin MA, Barfod C. New clinical guidelines on the spinal stabilisation of adult trauma patients–consensus and evidence based. Scand J Trauma Resusc Emerg Med. 2019;27(1):1–10.

Meyer JP, Barrett JA, Schuler JJ, et al. Mandatory versus selective exploration for penetrating neck trauma. A prospective assessment. Arch Surg. 1987;122:592–7.

Mohan B, Singal S, Bawa AS, Mahindra P, Yamin M. Endovascular management of traumatic pseudoaneurysm: short & long term outcomes. J Clin Orthop Trauma. 2017;8(3):276–80.

Mueller CA, Peters I, Podlogar M, Kovacs A, Urbach H, Schaller K, Schramm J, Kral T. Vertebral artery injuries following cervical spine trauma: a prospective observational study. Eur Spine J. 2011;20(12):2202–9.

Muralidhar BM, Hegde D, Hussain PS. Management of unstable thoracolumbar spinal fractures by pedicle screws and rods fixation. J Clin Diagn Res. 2014;8(2):121.

Nowicki JL, Stew B, Ooi E. Penetrating neck injuries: a guide to evaluation and management. Ann R Coll Surg Engl. 2017;100(1):6–11.

Phang I, Papadopoulos MC. Intraspinal pressure monitoring in a patient with spinal cord injury reveals different intradural compartments: injured spinal cord pressure evaluation (ISCoPE) study. Neurocrit Care. 2015;23(3):414–8.

Przybylski GJ. Management of odontoid fractures. Contemp Neurosurg. 1998;20:1–6.

Pulivarthi S, Gurram MK. Effectiveness of d-dimer as a screening test for venous thromboembolism: an update. N Am J Med Sci. 2014;6(10):491.

Radvany MG, Murphy KJ, Millward SF, Barr JD, Clark TW, Halin NJ, Kinney TB, Kundu S, Sacks D, Wallace MJ, Cardella JF. Research reporting standards for percutaneous vertebral augmentation. J Vasc Interv Radiol. 2009;20(10):1279–86.

Rajasekaran S, Kanna RM, Shetty AP. Management of thoracolumbar spine trauma: an overview. Indian J Orthop. 2015;49(1):72.

Riascos R, Bonfante E, Cotes C, Guirguis M, Hakimelahi R, West C. Imaging of atlantooccipital and atlantoaxial traumatic injuries: what the radiologist needs to know. Radiographics. 2015;35(7):2121–34.

Rozzelle CJ, Aarabi B, Dhall SS, et al. Management of pediatric cervical spine and spinal cord injuries. Neurosurgery. 2013;72(Suppl 2):205–26.

Sabiston CP, Wing PC. Sacral fractures: classification and neurologic implications. J Trauma. 1986;26:1113–5.

Shahlaie K, Chang DJ, Anderson JT. Nonmissile penetrating spinal injury: case report and review of the literature. J Neurosurg Spine. 2006;4(5):400–8.

Singh RR, Barry MC, Ireland A, et al. Current diagnosis and management of blunt internal carotid artery injury. Eur J Vasc Endovasc Surg. 2004;27(6):577–84.

Sözen T, Özışık L, Başaran NÇ. An overview and management of osteoporosis. Eur J Rheumatol. 2017;4(1):46.

Statements PC. Prevention of venous thromboembolism in individuals with spinal cord injury: clinical practice guidelines for health care providers. Top Spinal Cord Inj Rehabil. 2016;22(3):209–40.

Suss RA, Zimmerman RD, Leeds NE. Pseudospread of the atlas: false sign of Jefferson fracture in young children. AJR. 1983;140:1079–82.

Tannoury C, Degiacomo A. Fatal vertebral artery injury in penetrating cervical spine trauma. Case Rep Neurol Med. 2015;12:2015.

Theodore N, Aarabi B, Dhall SS, et al. The diagnosis and management of traumatic atlanto-occipital dislocation injuries. Neurosurgery. 2013a;72(Suppl 2):114–26.

Theodore N, et al. Occipital condyle fractures. Neurosurgery. 2013b;72:106–13.

Vaccaro AR, Lehman RA Jr, Hurlbert RJ, et al. A new classification of thoracolumbar injuries: the importance of injury morphology, the integrity of the posterior ligamentous complex, and neurologic status. Spine. 2005;30:2325–33.

Wasner G, Schattschneider J, Binder A, Baron R. Complex regional pain syndrome–diagnostic, mechanisms, CNS involvement and therapy. Spinal Cord. 2003;41(2):61–75.

Wilson JR, Cadotte DW, Fehlings MG. Clinical predictors of neurological outcome, functional status, and survival after traumatic spinal cord injury: a systematic review. J Neurosurg Spine. 2012;17(1, Suppl):11–26.

Zaveri G, Das G. Management of sub-axial cervical spine injuries. Indian J Orthop. 2017;51:633–52.

Complications, Outcomes, and Other Aspects

Eleni D-Tsianaka, Mohammed A. Al-Rawi,
Ruqayah A. Al-baidar, Mustafa M. Altaweel,
Mohammed A. Al-Dhahir, Zahraa F. Al-Sharshahi,
Ali A. Dolachee, and Samer S. Hoz

Contents

Suggested Reading – 129

S. S. Hoz et al., *Neurotrauma*, https://doi.org/10.1007/978-3-030-80869-3_6

1. Post-traumatic syringomyelia (PTS).
The *FALSE* answer is:
A. A cystic cavitation within the spinal cord.
B. Develops within 5 years of spinal cord injury (SCI).
C. Excellent outcomes after initial surgery.
D. Has a prevalence of 4%.
E. Rare complication of SCI.

Answer C
- PTS is associated with worsening symptoms over several years. Patients with PTS typically have unfavorable long-term outcomes. More than half of patients would require re-surgery.
- Symptoms of PTS are pain, numbness, or increased weakness.

6

2. PTS.
The *FALSE* answer is:
A. 68% of cases treated conservatively will deteriorate with time.
B. Most commonly develops after cervical spine injury.
C. Occurs more often to patients with complete quadriplegia.
D. Cordectomy is a surgical option only in syringomyelia with complete spinal cord injury.
E. Syringo-subarachnoid shunt has good results for pain relief.

Answer B
- Post-traumatic syringomyelia is more likely to develop after thoracic spine injury.

3. Delayed cervical instability.
The *FALSE* answer is:
A. Diagnosed at least 20 days after the injury.
B. Cervical muscles spasm can temporarily present the injury as stable.
C. Cervical vertebrae microfractures are not implicated.
D. There is no model to predict it.
E. Cervical spine subluxations <3 mm should be re-evaluated.

Answer C
- Microfractures, spasm of the cervical muscles, and positioning of the patient during initial imaging are some of the reasons for early instability recognition failure.

❓ 4. Delayed deterioration.

The *FALSE* answer is:

A. Formation of scar tissue can cause tethered spinal cord syndrome.

B. Glial scar formation does not play a role in neuro-regenerative failure.

C. The mean time for appearance of symptoms of post-traumatic syringomyelia is 9 years.

D. Neuronal cell apoptosis can last for years.

E. Spinal epidural hematoma can occur after the first 72 h post-operatively.

✅ Answer B

— Glial scar formation can cause failure to the neuro-regenerative process by acting as a physical barrier and also by also due to the inhibitory nature of it's cellular and molecular components.

❓ 5. Post-traumatic spasticity.

The *FALSE* answer is:

A. May present months after the injury.

B. Ashworth score: grade 3: considerable increase in muscle tone, passive movements difficult.

C. Diazepam is most beneficial in patients with complete spinal cord injuries.

D. CSF collection is a complication of intra-thecal baclofen pump.

E. Severe intra-thecal baclofen withdrawal syndrome can cause rhabdomyolysis.

✅ Answer B

— "Considerable increase muscle tone, passive movements difficult" is considered as grade 4.

— "More marked increase muscle tone, passive movements easy" is considered as grade 3.

— Severe intra-thecal baclofen withdrawal syndrome can cause rhabdomyolysis, hepatic and renal failure, even death.

❓ 6. Spinal CSF leak.

The *FALSE* answer is:

A. Spinal trauma is the most common cause.

B. Dural tears are more common in thoracic spine trauma.

C. Steroid administration can increase the risk of CSF leak.

D. Lumbar drain can cause infections.

E. Lumbar drain over-drainage can lead to brainstem compression.

✔️ **Answer A**

— Spinal trauma is a rare cause of CSF leak.

❓ **7. Spinal CSF leak.**

The *FALSE* answer is:

A. Severe postural headache is a common symptom.

B. Beta 2-transferin in the suspected fluid is diagnostic.

C. Bed rest and lumbar drain are the first-line treatment.

D. Epidural blood patch can be effective in up to 67–75% of the cases.

E. Open surgery is the first-line treatment.

6

✔️ **Answer E**

— Surgery is the last choice, after all conservative and minimal invasive measures fail.

— Severe postural headache, neck stiffness, and tenderness are common symptoms.

❓ **8. Deep vein thrombosis (DVT).**

The *FALSE* answer is:

A. 50–60% of patients initially do not present typically.

B. Incidence of DVT approaches 100% when 125I-fibrinogen is used.

C. Vena cava interruption filters used as routine prophylaxis.

D. Side effects of heparin include thrombosis and thrombocytopenia.

E. The mortality rate is 9%.

✔️ **Answer C**

— Vena cava interruption filters are not indicated for routine prophylaxis; they may be used for candidate patients who fail anticoagulation or where anticoagulation cannot be used.

— Side effects of heparin include thrombosis, thrombocytopenia, and osteoporosis on long-term use.

❓ **9. Post-traumatic spine deformity.**

The *FALSE* answer is:

A. Thoracolumbar burst fractures: conservative treatment require regular X-rays.

B. Thoracolumbar burst fractures: progressive kyphosis is an indication for surgery.
C. Lumbar compression fractures: progressive kyphosis less likely than thoracic.
D. Lumbar compression fractures with >75% decrease in anterior vertebral body: increased risk for progressive kyphosis.
E. Isolated posterior column disruption may develop into a progressive kyphotic deformity.

✅ **Answer C**
- Compression fractures of the lumbar spine are more likely to develop progressive kyphosis, than those of the thoracic spine.

❓ **10. Infections.**
The *FALSE* answer is:
A. Urinary tract infection is the second most common cause of death.
B. Asymptomatic bacteriuria is not an indication for systemic antibiotic therapy.
C. Patients with cervical spinal cord injury are less likely to develop pneumonia.
D. Poor nutrition is a predisposing factor for pressure ulcers.
E. High levels of plasma fibronectin are associated with improved ulcer healing.

✅ **Answer C**
- Cervical spinal cord injury can lead to difficulties with normal coughing; thus, these patients are more likely to develop pneumonia.

❓ **11. Respiratory complications.**
The *FALSE* answer is:
A. Respiratory failure is most common during the acute phase.
B. Pleural effusion is not common.
C. Tetraplegic patients have higher risk of pneumonia.
D. Suctioning must be avoided.
E. Pneumococcal vaccine is recommended.

✅ Answer D
- Suctioning is a prevention measure for respiratory complications.
- Routine vaccinations for influenza and pneumococcal infections are recommended.

❓ 12. Osteoporosis.
The _FALSE_ answer is:
A. Patients are more prone to vitamin D deficiency.
B. Patients with elevated serum calcium levels must reduce daily calcium intake.
C. Bisphosphonates are a treatment option.
D. Teriparatide can stimulate osteoblast activity.
E. Patients with complete SCI lose up to 1% of bone mineral density per week.

✅ Answer B
- Even when serum calcium levels are increased, patients must not reduce the daily calcium intake, because the parathyroid hormone is suppressed, decreasing the calcium absorption.

❓ 13. Heterotopic ossifications (HO).
The _FALSE_ answer is:
A. Most common at the hips and knees.
B. Associated with increased levels of alkaline phosphatase.
C. Patients with complete spinal cord injury are more susceptible.
D. Nonsteroidal anti-inflammatories are more effective as prophylaxis than as treatment.
E. Radiotherapy is an instigating factor.

✅ Answer E
- Radiotherapy is an option for prophylaxis and treatment for HO.

❓ 14. CSF fistula after spinal gun shot.
The _FALSE_ answer is:
A. May occur at entrance or exit site.
B. Subarachnoid drainage is not advised.
C. Prophylactic antibiotics decrease the incidence of infection.
D. Connection to pleural cavity may occur.
E. Surgical exploration is warranted if other measures fail.

✅ **Answer B**
- The primary management of CSF fistula should be with subarachnoid drainage. If this fails, surgical exploration is necessary.
- Connection to bowel, bladder, or pleural cavity may occur.

❓ **15. Spinal gunshot foreign body related complications.**
The *FALSE* answer is:
A. Migration in a symptomatic patient is an indication for surgery.
B. Lead intoxication is common.
C. Symptomatic neural compression warrants surgical removal of the bullet.
D. Removal does not improve deafferentation pain.
E. If left, will become encapsulated by poorly vascularized fibrous tissue.

✅ **Answer B**
- Lead intoxication is rare.

❓ **16. Vascular injury during cervical spine surgery.**
The *FALSE* answer is:
A. Vertebral artery (VA) may be injured in posterior approaches to C1-C2.
B. Vertebral artery (VA) is not at risk in anterior approaches to the subaxial cervical spine.
C. Carotid artery may be injured in anterior cervical discectomy and fusion (ACDF).
D. If vertebral artery repair is unattainable, ligation should be done.
E. In cases of vascular injury, postoperative angiography is indicated.

✅ **Answer B**
- VA can be injured in anterior subaxial cervical approaches. The VA runs anterior to the ventral rami of the cervical nerves from C2 to C6 and may be injured during to mechanized air drilling, screw tapping, and soft tissue retraction.

17. Complications that can be recognized intraoperatively.
The *FALSE* answer is:
A. Pedicle breach.
B. Dural tear.
C. Vascular injury.
D. Facet violation.
E. Pseudoarthrosis.

Answer E
- Pseudoarthrosis can only be recognised postoperatively. Asymptomatic patients may be followed for the development of any problems. Symptomatic nonunions may require repair, but careful diagnostic workup is necessary to rule out other sources of symptoms (e.g., adjacent level disease and stenosis).
- All the other options are possible to be recognized intraoperatively as well as postoperatively.

6

18. Spine kyphotic deformity after trauma.
The *FALSE* answer is:
A. A sagittal plane deformity.
B. Caused primarily by a distraction-extension mechanism.
C. More common than lordotic deformity.
D. More common in the thoracolumbar junction.
E. Anterior decompression and posterior segmental stabilization are options.

Answer B
- Kyphotic deformity is generally caused by a flexion- or compression-type injury.
- Lordotic deformity may be seen following a primarily distraction-extension mechanism with disruption of the anterior longitudinal ligament, intervertebral disc complex, and compromise to the osseous posterior elements.

19. Translational spine injury.
The *FALSE* answer is:
A. Dramatic instability of the vertebral column.
B. May be caused by a shear-type injury.
C. May be caused by a combined-type injury.

D. Spares the posterior column.
E. Requires multiple-approach surgical therapy.

✅ **Answer D**

— Translational deformities are caused by a shear type or combined injury mechanism and often lead to dramatic instability of the vertebral column due to injury to all three spinal columns.

Suggested Reading

Agarwal NK, Mathur N. Deep vein thrombosis in acute spinal cord injury. Spinal Cord. 2009;47(10):769–72.

Bauman WA, Cardozo CP. Osteoporosis in individuals with spinal cord injury. PM R. 2015;7(2):188–201. https://doi.org/10.1016/j.pmrj.2014.08.948.

Baunsgaard CB, Nissen UV, Christensen KB, Biering-Sørensen F. Modified Ashworth scale and spasm frequency score in spinal cord injury: reliability and correlation. Spinal Cord. 2016;54(9):702–8.

Beutel WE, Roberts JD, Langston HT, et al. Subarachnoid-pleural fistula. J Thorac Cardiovasc Surg. 1980;80:21–4.

Carroll ÁM, Brackenridge P. Post-traumatic syringomyelia: a review of the cases presenting in a regional spinal injuries unit in the north east of England over a 5-year period. Spine. 2005;30(10):1206–10.

Elsissy J, Kutzner A, Danisa O. Delayed diagnosis and management of traumatic cervical spine subluxation. J Orthop Case Rep. 2019;9(4):84.

Harrop JS, Sharan AD, Vaccaro AR, Przybylski GJ. The cause of neurologic deterioration after acute cervical spinal cord injury. Spine. 2001;26(4):340–6.

Khurana B, Sheehan SE, Sodickson A, Bono CM, Harris MB. Traumatic thoracolumbar spine injuries: what the spine surgeon wants to know. Radiographics. 2013;33(7):2031–46.

Kim HG, San Oh H, Kim TW, Park KH. Clinical features of post-traumatic Syringomyelia. Korean J Neurotrauma. 2014;10(2):66.

Lee SE, Chung CK, Jahng TA, Kim CH. Dural tear and resultant cerebrospinal fluid leaks after cervical spinal trauma. Eur Spine J. 2014;23(8):1772–6.

Łęgosz P, Drela K, Pulik Ł, Sarzyńska S, Małdyk P. Challenges of heterotopic ossification – molecular background and current treatment strategies. Clin Exp Pharmacol Physiol. 2018;45(12):1229–35. https://doi.org/10.1111/1440-1681.13025.

Leven D, Cho SK. Pseudarthrosis of the cervical spine: risk factors, diagnosis and management. Asian Spine J. 2016;10(4):776.

Lunardini DJ, Eskander MS, Even JL, Dunlap JT, Chen AF, Lee JY, Ward TW, Kang JD, Donaldson WF. Vertebral artery injuries in cervical spine surgery. Spine J. 2014;14(8):1520–5.

Munting E. Surgical treatment of post-traumatic kyphosis in the thoracolumbar spine: indications and technical aspects. Eur Spine J. 2010;19(1):69–73.

Oh JW, Kim SH, Whang K. Traumatic cerebrospinal fluid leak: diagnosis and management. Korean J Neurotrauma. 2017;13(2):63.

Sezer N, Akkus S, Ugurlu FG. Chronic complications of spinal cord injury. World J Orthop. 2015;6(1):24–33.

Siroky MB. Pathogenesis of bacteriuria and infection in the spinal cord injured patient. Am J Med. 2002;113(Suppl 1A):67S–79S.

Vaccaro AR, Silber JS. Post-traumatic spinal deformity. Spine. 2001;26(24S):S111–8.

Ward WE, Maltby GL. Associated complications in war wounds of the spine. JAMA. 1945;129:155–7.

6

Peripheral Neurotrauma and Miscellaneous Issues

Contents

Chapter 7   Peripheral Nerve Neurotrauma – 133

Chapter 8   Miscellaneous Issues Related
to Neurotrauma – 149

Peripheral Nerve Neurotrauma

Rasha A. Alshakarchy, Mustafa Qusai Saoodi, Elena Nestian, Laith Thamir Al-Ameri, Ghazwan Hazim Albu-Salih, Mohammed K. Alaskari, Awfa A. Aktham, Sama S. Albairmani, Zahraa F. Al-Sharshahi, and Samer S. Hoz

Contents

Suggested Reading – 146

© The Author(s), under exclusive license to Springer Nature Switzerland AG 2022
S. S. Hoz et al., *Neurotrauma*, https://doi.org/10.1007/978-3-030-80869-3_7

? 1. **Anatomy**
   The _FALSE_ answer is:
   A. Oligodendrocytes produce myelin in peripheral nervous system (PNS).
   B. Axon is the basic unit of a peripheral nerve.
   C. Epineurium surrounds the main nerve trunk.
   D. Perineurium surrounds the nerve fascicle.
   E. Endoneurium surrounds the axons.

✔ **Answer A**
   ▬ Schwann cells produce the myelin in PNS, whereas the oligodendrocytes produce myelin in CNS.

? 2. **Seddon classification.**
   The _FALSE_ answer is:
   A. Neuropraxia means conduction block.
   B. Neuropraxia involves the myelin only.
   C. Axonotmesis is also known as neuroma-in-continuity.
   D. Axonotmesis involves the epineurium.
   E. Neurotmesis involves the disruption of all nerve layers.

✔ **Answer D**
   ▬ Axonotmesis involves disruption of the myelin and the axon with intact epineurium.

? 3. **Sunderland classification Grade I.**
   The _FALSE_ answer is:
   A. Equals neuropraxia.
   B. Involves loss of myelin only.
   C. Autonomic function is usually not affected.
   D. Recovery is dismal.
   E. Duration of recovery is from 1 to 4 months.

✔ **Answer D**
   ▬ Excellent recovery is expected with conservative management within 1–4 months.

7

❓ 4. Sunderland classification, Grade II.
   The *FALSE* answer is:
   A. Axonal loss.
   B. Preserved endoneurium.
   C. Loss of autonomic function.
   D. Time of recovery dependent on the level of injury.
   E. Disrupted perineurium.

✔️ Answer E
   − Endoneurium, epineurium, and perineurium are preserved.
   − Axons extend along the intact endoneurium at a speed of 1–3 mm per day.

❓ 5. Sunderland classification, Grade III.
   The *FALSE* answer is:
   A. Disrupted endoneurium.
   B. Injured perineurium.
   C. Intact nerve fascicle.
   D. High rate of scar formation.
   E. Axon rerouting.

✔️ Answer B
   − Intact perineurium, the fascicles are preserved as tubes, but their insides are damaged.
   − The scars created can cause rerouting of the regenerating axons not reaching their original targets, which is more evident for mixed nerves (motor and sensory).

❓ 6. Sunderland classification, Grade IV.
   The *FALSE* answer is:
   A. Intact perineurium.
   B. Undamaged epineurium.
   C. Disrupted fascicles.
   D. Little or no recovery.
   E. Treated surgically.

◘ Table 7.1   Sunderland classification of nerve injuries

Classification of nerve injuries				
Sunderland **I**	**II**	**III**	**IV**	**V**
Focal conduction block No Wallerian degeneration	Axonal disruption	Axon + Endoneurium disruption	Axon + Endoneurium + Perineurium disruption	Axon + Endoneurium + Perineurium + epineurium disruption

✔ Answer A
- The perineurium is disrupted in grade 4 (**◘** Table 7.1).

❓ 7. Sunderland classification, Grade V.
The *FALSE* answer is:
A. Partially or completely severed nerve.
B. Equals neurotmesis.
C. Involvement of endoneurium, perineurium, and epineurium.
D. Caused by avulsion injuries.
E. Approached surgically.

✔ Answer D
- Commonly caused by laceration injuries.

❓ 8. Sunderland classification, clinical relevance.
The *FALSE* answer is:
A. Correlates with the clinical picture.
B. Describes the extent of injury.
C. Describes treatment modalities.
D. Dictates specific surgical management.
E. Provides prognostic information.

✔ Answer D
- The Sunderland classification indicates whether the injury should be managed surgically or conservatively, but it has no role in determining the surgical intervention (**◘** Table 7.2).

◘ **Table 7.2** Sunderland Classification

Injury grade	Patho-anatomy	Recovery potential
I	Localized segmental demyelination	Spontaneous complete days-weeks
II	Axon injury with Wallerian degeneration	Full recovery possible without surgery at 2–3 mm/day
III	Axon and endoneurium disrupted	Spontaneous incomplete recovery 1 mm/day
IV	Perineurium disrupted	Surgical reconstruction required with resection and graft anticipated recovery incomplete
V	Epineurium disrupted	Surgical reconstruction necessary with resection and graft anticipated recovery incomplete

9. Pathophysiology of nerve injury.
The *FALSE* answer is:
A. Neurotropism is a chemotactic gradient that attracts a regenerating axon toward the target.
B. Neurotropism is the nutritional support provided to axons connecting with the stump.
C. Wallerian degeneration is the degeneration of the distal nerve stump.
D. Chromatolysis is the axonal degeneration distal to the injury.
E. A neuroma is a "confused" nerve ending resulting in pain and dysfunction.

✔ **Answer D**
━ Chromatolysis is the process by which axonal degeneration occurs proximal to the injury.

10. Two-point sensory discrimination.
The *FALSE* answer is:
A. 6 mm represents a normal static two-point discrimination.
B. 3 mm represents a normal dynamic two-point discrimination.
C. It is most applicable for nerve injuries.
D. It is less reliable in compression neuropathies.
E. Semmes-Weinstein monofilaments are used.

✅ **Answer E**

 ▬ Semmes-Weinstein monofilaments are not used for two-point discrimination. They are used to measure pressure thresholds and are most applicable to compression neuropathies, as well as complete nerve injuries.

❓ **11. Lesions in continuity.**
   The _FALSE_ answer is:
   A. Caused by traction injuries.
   B. Retraction and scarring are common.
   C. Always Grade I Sunderland injuries.
   D. Focal or diffuse.
   E. Improve over time.

✅ **Answer C**

Lesions in continuity
 ▬ Can be any grade in Sunderland classification.
 ▬ Can improve over time; re-evaluation is recommended after several months.
 ▬ Caused by stretch, traction, or contusion.

❓ **12. Avulsion injury.**
   The _FALSE_ answer is:
   A. Brachial plexus injury is the least common.
   B. All grades of damage can occur.
   C. May be associated with vascular injury.
   D. Spinal nerves are injured in the gutter of the transverse process.
   E. Delayed surgical exploration is performed.

✅ **Answer A**

 ▬ Brachial plexus injury is the most common.
 ▬ These types of injuries pose a difficult challenge, as there may not be a satisfactory operative solution for most of them.

❓ **13. Compartment injury.**
   The _FALSE_ answer is:
   A. Medical emergency.
   B. Caused by severe crush injuries.
   C. Ischemic necrosis occurs in peripheral nerves.
   D. The most common is median nerve compartment syndrome.
   E. Repair of the necrotic segment can be easily achieved.

✅ **Answer E**
- The necrotic segment is often long, making surgical repair unrealistic.
- Immediate fasciotomy is required to halt the process of ischemia and subsequent necrosis.
- Caused by severe crush injuries with skeletal fractures and vascular compromise.
- The most common is median nerve compartment syndrome due to brachial artery injury.

❓ **14. Rare forms of injury.**
   The *FALSE* answer is:
   A. Injection injury is related only to the needle puncture.
   B. Injection injury mostly involves the sciatic nerve.
   C. Radiation injury mostly involves brachial plexus.
   D. Thermal injury is either direct or secondary to constrictive fibrosis.
   E. Electrical injury produces long segments of necrotic non-functioning nerves.

✅ **Answer A**
- Injection injury results from damage caused by the needle puncture and more commonly from the toxic effect of the injected material; it depends on the site of injection (inside or close to the nerve).
- Radiation injury is often dose-dependent, symptoms may start months to years following treatment, due to extensive fibrosis and axonal degeneration.

❓ **15. Nerve conduction studies and EMG after axonal injury.**
   The *FALSE* answer is:
   A. Increased distal motor latency.
   B. Absent fibrillation potentials.
   C. Presence of positive sharp waves.
   D. Decreased amplitudes.
   E. Decreased conductive velocity.

✅ **Answer B**
- Fibrillation potentials are seen in axonal injury.

❓ **16. Electro-diagnostic studies (EDSs).**
   The *FALSE* answer is:
   A. Wallerian degeneration (WD) is complete after 3 weeks of trauma.

B. EDSs should be performed before WD is complete.
C. EDSs are indicated after 3 weeks of trauma.
D. EDSs can identify the site of injury accurately.
E. EDSs can assess progression and estimate prognosis.

✅ Answer B
- The optimal timing for EDSs to be performed is after WD is complete, as none of the electrical changes are evident earlier.
- Wallerian degeneration affects the distal axonal segments, cell bodies, or target organs; it starts immediately after injury and is completed only after 3 weeks.

❓ 17. Magnetic resonance neurography (MRN).
The *FALSE* answer is:
A. Neuropraxia shows increased nerve signal intensity on T2.
B. Neuropraxia shows mild muscular atrophy.
C. Axonotmesis and neurotmesis show signs of muscle denervation.
D. Axonotmesis shows enlarged nerve with loss of fascicular pattern.
E. Acute neurotmesis shows terminal neuroma.

✅ Answer E
- Chronic neurotmesis shows terminal neuroma, whereas acute neurotmesis shows nerve discontinuity, gap filled with fluid and granulation tissue with increased SI pattern on T2 Magnetic resonance neurography (MRN).

❓ 18. Ultrasonographic evaluation.
The *FALSE* answer is:
A. Uses high resolution ultrasound with restricted tissue penetration.
B. Provides morphological information of the injured segment.
C. Replaces MRN in the setting of osteosynthetic materials.
D. Surgical approach and skin incision can be precisely targeted.
E. Cannot distinguish between direct and indirect injuries.

✅ Answer E
- Ultrasonography can distinguish between direct (transection) and indirect injuries (compression secondary to scar tissue, osteosynthetic material, or hematoma).

❓ 19. Surgical intervention.
   The _FALSE_ answer is:
   A. Nerve stretching.
   B. Direct repair.
   C. Nerve graft.
   D. Nerve transfer.
   E. Nerve tube.

✅ Answer A
   – Nerve stretching, bone shortening, extremity positioning, and stump mobilization were some of the procedures used in the past to shorten the gap, which are now obsolete.

❓ 20. General surgical principles.
   The _FALSE_ answer is:
   A. Tension-free repair.
   B. Debridement up to healthy nerve tissue.
   C. Perfect fascicular alignment.
   D. Long-acting muscle relaxants are used.
   E. Atraumatic and secure mechanical approximation is used.

✅ Answer D
   – Short-acting muscle relaxant must be used if intraoperative stimulation is needed to test for muscle contraction; otherwise, such tests are inapplicable with muscle relaxant use.

❓ 21. Neurolysis.
   The _FALSE_ answer is:
   A. External neurolysis entails dissection outside the epineurium.
   B. Enables mobilization of the nerve.
   C. Performed from the injured site toward the normal tissue.
   D. Provides sufficient exposure of the injured segment.
   E. Adequate neurolysis improves vascularity.

✅ Answer C
   – Neurolysis entails epineural release from compression points or tethering by fibrosis; it is preferably performed toward the injured site starting from a normal nerve segment.

7

? 22. Direct nerve repair.
   The *FALSE* answer is:
   A. Indicated when there is minimal gap.
   B. Better results for mixed nerves.
   C. Tension-free repair is the principle.
   D. End-to-end repair includes epineural or fascicular repair.
   E. End-to-side repair is particularly useful for sensory and facial nerves.

✓ Answer B
   – Better outcomes are observed in exclusively motor or sensory nerves.
   – Acceptable tension is poorly defined, but failure to hold an end-to-end repair with a single suture (using 9-0 suture) is a sign of excessive tension.

? 23. Nerve grafts.
   The *FALSE* answer is:
   A. Indicated for gaps less than 2 cm.
   B. Sural nerve is the most frequent autograft used.
   C. Fibrin glue may be used.
   D. Fewer sutures are recommended to avoid fibrosis.
   E. Allografts require immunosuppressants.

✓ Answer A
   – Indicated for gaps more than 3 cm.
   – Allografts require tissue matching and immunosuppressive therapy.
   – Autografts are the gold standard, but complications include donor site neurological deficit, additional incision, wound complications, limited availability, neuroma formation, and neuropathic pain.

? 24. Nerve tubes.
   The *FALSE* answer is:
   A. Involve the use of non-nerve graft as a conduit for axonal regeneration.
   B. Indicated for short gaps (less than 3 cm).
   C. Tube diameter is the same as nerve diameter.
   D. Ideally, the tube should be biodegradable.
   E. Autologous grafts are superior to artificial ones.

✓ Answer C
   – Tube diameter should be 20% more than the nerve diameter, because tubes tend to swell and compress the neural elements.

- Autologous tubes include inside-out veins and arteries, tendons, skeletal muscles, epineural sheaths, and human amniotic membranes.

? 25. A 4 cm gap of the ulnar nerve above the elbow.
The *FALSE* answer is:
A. Anterior transposition of the nerve to gain length is a possibility.
B. One sural nerve would provide sufficient cable graft for this defect.
C. This is a good indication for a vascularized nerve transfer.
D. Neurotization is usually associated with inferior functional outcome compared to grafting.
E. This defect is large enough to justify the use of a synthetic conduit.

✓ Answer C
- Vascularized nerve grafts are generally reserved for extensively scarred tissues, such as tissues that have undergone radiotherapy.

? 26. One week after digital nerve injury by sharp division.
The *FALSE* answer is:
A. A direct repair should still be possible at this stage.
B. Fascicular repair would give an equivalent result to epineurial repair.
C. An 8 mm deficit is better repaired with a nerve graft.
D. Trimming the nerve ends should be avoided to preserve length.
E. The injured site should be splinted after repair.

✓ Answer D
- Bulging fascicles should be trimmed to allow a neat epineurial repair.

? 27. Gunshot injuries.
The *FALSE* answer is:
A. Produce lesions in continuity.
B. When potential for spontaneous recovery, exploration is delayed for 3 to 4 months.
C. Association with vascular injury is an indication for emergent surgical exploration.
D. Lower brachial plexus injuries are treated conservatively, except in resistant non-causalgic pain.
E. In sciatic nerve injuries, peroneal division repair is the priority.

✓ Answer E
- In sciatic nerve injuries, tibial division repair is the priority.

② 28. Gunshot high radial nerve injury.
   The *FALSE* answer is:
   A. Immediate surgical exploration is performed.
   B. Re-exploration is recommended if no recovery is seen on EMG 2 months after injury.
   C. Suture tagging of nerve stumps is performed.
   D. Good soft tissue cover is aimed.
   E. Nerve trimming is performed.

✓ Answer B
   ▬ Re-exploration is indicated if no recovery is seen on electromyography (EMG) 3–6 months following the injury.

② 29. Postoperative care.
   The *FALSE* answer is:
   A. Early mobilization and extensive physiotherapy are encouraged.
   B. Adequate hemostasis should be achieved.
   C. Suction drains are avoided.
   D. Bulky dressing and padding are used.
   E. Shoulder immobilization by sling is performed after brachial plexus repair.

✓ Answer A
   ▬ The strength of a nerve repair usually plateaus after 3 weeks; hence, movement is restricted for that period with gradual physiotherapy and exercise beyond that time.

② 30. Timing of surgery.
   The *FALSE* answer is:
   A. Sharp lacerations are best treated within the first 72 hours of injury.
   B. Blunt lacerations are best explored after 3 to 4 weeks of injury.
   C. Closed injuries are best explored after 3 to 4 days of injury.
   D. Gunshot wounds are best treated conservatively from 4 to 6 months after injury.
   E. Nerve surgery should be avoided when the duration of the total muscle denervation exceeds 18 to 24 months.

✓ Answer C
   ▬ Closed injuries are best explored after 3 to 4 months following injury. Except for closed injuries with acute nerve compression, which should be evaluated and explored urgently.

❓ 31. Outcomes following nerve injury.
The *FALSE* answer is:
A. Peripheral and central nerve injury outcomes are broadly different.
B. Median nerve repairs tend to gain superior results to those of the ulnar nerve.
C. Excision of a neuroma is best carried out early, about 6 weeks after repair.
D. Inter-positional autologous nerve grafts give poor results in motor nerve repair.
E. After an initial delay, nerve recovery occurs at approximately 1 inch per month.

✅ Answer C
— A neuroma may not be evident at 6 weeks and there may be other reasons for pain and irritation at the site of repair at this early stage, such as scar hypersensitivity.

❓ 32. Prognosis.
The *FALSE* answer is:
A. Earlier initiation of regeneration.
B. Increased rate of neuronal regeneration.
C. Greater stability of the neuromuscular junction after denervation.
D. Better in longer extremities.
E. Increased adaptability of effector muscles to substitute their function.

✅ Answer D
— Shorter extremities. The prognosis is better in younger patients.

❓ 33. Prognosis, regarding injured nerve characteristics.
The *FALSE* answer is:
A. Better in pure nerves than combined.
B. Better in pure sensory than in pure motor nerves.
C. Better in oligo-fascicular nerves.
D. Better in highly vascularized nerves.
E. Worse in nerves with bulky intraneural connective tissue.

✅ Answer B
— The prognosis is worse in pure sensory than in pure motor nerves.

❓ 34. Prognosis, regarding main muscle effector characteristics.
The *FALSE* answer is:
A. Better if functional recovery can be acquired with fewer nerve fibers.
B. Better if complete muscle strength is not necessary for function.
C. Better for distally innervated muscles.
D. Better if other muscles can compensate for loss of function.
E. Better if not necessary to restore precise or coordinated muscle function.

✅ Answer C
— Better for the muscles that receive the innervation proximally.

❓ 35. Prognosis, regarding nerve injury.
The *FALSE* answer is:
A. Mechanism of injury, better in traction injuries.
B. Depends on the severity of trauma.
C. Level of injury, better for distal nerve injuries.
D. Time after trauma, good before muscle atrophy has occurred.
E. Length of injured nerve, better for shorter segments involved.

✅ Answer A
— The prognosis is better in lacerations and worse in traction or missile injuries.
— Muscle atrophy starts within 3 weeks of denervation with almost complete replacement of the muscle with fibrous tissue over the next 2 years.

Suggested Reading

Akhavan-Sigari R, Mielke D, Farhadi A, Rohde V. Study of radial nerve injury caused by gunshot wounds and explosive injuries among Iraqi soldiers. Open Access Maced J Med Sci. 2018;6(9):1622.

Ali ZS, Pisapia JM, Ma TS, Zager EL, Heuer GG, Khoury V. Ultrasonographic evaluation of peripheral nerves. World Neurosurg. 2016;85:333–9.

Carlstedt T. New treatments for spinal nerve root avulsion injury. Front Neurol. 2016;7:135.

Carter GT, Robinson LR, Chang VH, Kraft GH. Electrodiagnostic evaluation of traumatic nerve injuries. Hand Clin. 2000;16(1):1–2.

Chehrazi B. Peripheral nerve injuries: principles of surgical management and outcome. J Neurotrauma. 1989;6(3):191–6.

Chen SL, Chen ZG, Dai HL, Ding JX, Guo JS, Han N, Jiang BG, Jiang HJ, Li J, Li SP, Li WJ. Repair, protection and regeneration of peripheral nerve injury. Neural Regen Res. 2015;10(11):1777.

Chhabra A, Ahlawat S, Belzberg A, Andreseik G. Peripheral nerve injury grading simplified on MR neurography: as referenced to Seddon and Sunderland classifications. Indian J Radiol Imaging. 2014;24(3):217.

Chichkova RI, Katzin L. EMG and nerve conduction studies in clinical practice. Pract Neurol. 2010;1(2010):32–8.

Deumens R, Bozkurt A, Meek MF, Marcus MA, Joosten EA, Weis J, Brook GA. Repairing injured peripheral nerves: bridging the gap. Prog Neurobiol. 2010;92(3):245–76.

Grant GA, Goodkin R, Kliot M. Evaluation and surgical management of peripheral nerve problems. Neurosurgery. 1999;44(4):825–39.

Griffin MF, Malahias M, Hindocha S, Khan WS. Peripheral nerve injury: principles for repair and regeneration. Open Orthop J. 2014;8:199–203.

He B, Zhu Z, Zhu Q, Zhou X, Zheng C, Li P, Zhu S, Liu X, Zhu J. Factors predicting sensory and motor recovery after the repair of upper limb peripheral nerve injuries. Neural Regen Res. 2014;9(6):661.

Heriseanu R, Baguley IJ, Slewa-Younan S. Two-point discrimination following traumatic brain injury. J Clin Neurosci. 2005;12(2):156–60.

Ichihara S, Inada Y, Nakamura T. Artificial nerve tubes and their application for repair of peripheral nerve injury: an update of current concepts. Injury. 2008;39:29–39.

Jia X, Romero-Ortega MI, Teng YD. Peripheral nerve regeneration: mechanism, cell biology, and therapies. Biomed Res Int. 2014;2014:145304.

Kornfeld T, Vogt PM, Radtke C. Nerve grafting for peripheral nerve injuries with extended defect sizes. Wien Med Wochenschr. 2019;169(9):240–51.

Lee SK, Wolfe SW. Peripheral nerve injury and repair. J Am Acad Orthop Surg. 2000;8(4):243–52.

Martins RS, Bastos D, Siqueira MG, Heise CO, Teixeira MJ. Traumatic injuries of peripheral nerves: a review with emphasis on surgical indication. Arq Neuropsiquiatr. 2013;71(10):811–4.

Menorca RM, Fussell TS, Elfar JC. Peripheral nerve trauma: mechanisms of injury and recovery. Hand Clin. 2013;29(3):317.

Mermans JF, Franssen BB, Serroyen J, Hulst RR. Digital nerve injuries: a review of predictors of sensory recovery after microsurgical digital nerve repair. Hand. 2012;7(3):233–41.

Moon LD. Chromatolysis: do injured axons regenerate poorly when ribonucleases attack rough endoplasmic reticulum, ribosomes and RNA? Dev Neurobiol. 2018;78(10):1011–24.

Osborn CP, Schmidt AH. Management of acute compartment syndrome. J Am Acad Orthop Surg. 2020;28(3):e108–14.

Pannell WC, Heckmann N, Alluri RK, Sivasundaram L, Stevanovic M, Ghiassi A. Predictors of nerve injury after gunshot wounds to the upper extremity. Hand. 2017;12(5):501–6.

Robinson MD, Shannon S. Rehabilitation of peripheral nerve injuries. Phys Med Rehabil Clin. 2002;13(1):109–35.

Salzer JL, Zalc B. Myelination. Curr Biol. 2016;26(20):R971–5.

Seddon HJ. A classification of nerve injuries. Br Med J. 1942;2(4260):237.

Stonner MM, Mackinnon SE, Kaskutas V. Predictors of functional outcome after peripheral nerve injury and compression. J Hand Ther. 2020;34:369–75.

Sunderland SI. Nerves and nerve injuries. 2nd ed. Edinburgh: Churchill Livingstone; 1978.

Wang E, Inaba K, Byerly S, Escamilla D, Cho J, Carey J, Stevanovic M, Ghiassi A, Demetriades D. Optimal timing for repair of peripheral nerve injuries. J Trauma Acute Care Surg. 2017;83(5):875–81.

Woo A, Bakri K, Moran SL. Management of ulnar nerve injuries. J Hand Surg Am. 2015;40(1):173–81.

Zuniga JR, Mistry C, Tikhonov I, Dessouky R, Chhabra A. Magnetic resonance neurography of traumatic and nontraumatic peripheral trigeminal neuropathies. J Oral Maxillofac Surg. 2018;76(4):725–36.

7

Miscellaneous Issues Related to Neurotrauma

Laith Thamir Al-Ameri, Hira Burhan, Mohammed A. Finjan, Mustapha Eyad, Zahraa M. Kareem, Zahraa A. Alsubaihawi, Ismail Al-Kebsi, Taha Mohammed Algahoom, Nawar Ghassan, Zahraa F. Al-Sharshahi, and Samer S. Hoz

Contents

Suggested Reading – 164

S. S. Hoz et al., *Neurotrauma*, https://doi.org/10.1007/978-3-030-80869-3_8

❓ 1. TBI. Child abuse.
   The *FALSE* answer is:
   A. Presents with specific history of trauma.
   B. Retinal hemorrhages.
   C. High mortality.
   D. Cerebral edema associated with poor outcomes.
   E. Subdural hematoma is common.

✅ Answer A
 ▬ Usually no specific history of trauma is given; the child may be brought in with different complaints such as drowsiness or even unconsciousness.

❓ 2. Shaken baby syndrome.
   The *FALSE* answer is:
   A. Retinal hemorrhage suggests the diagnosis of inflicted head injury.
   B. Outcome better than accidental head trauma.
   C. 95% of severe intracranial injuries are caused by abuse.
   D. Injury caused by translational or rotational forces.
   E. Retinal hemorrhage without subdural hemorrhage has not been reported.

✅ Answer B
 ▬ Morbidity and mortality outcomes are worse in inflicted brain trauma with the majority of survivors showing neurological or cognitive dysfunction later in life.

❓ 3. Mortality in polytrauma.
   The *FALSE* answer is:
   A. Brain injury is the leading cause of death.
   B. Immediate death (less than 1 hour): CNS and cardio vascular (CVS) injuries.
   C. Immediate mortality rate is up to 45% of victims.
   D. Early death (1 to 4 hours): multiple organ failure.
   E. Late death: systemic complications.

✅ Answer D
 ▬ CNS and CVS injuries are the predominant causes of both immediate and early death in polytrauma patients.

? 4. Acute abdomen associated with spinal cord injury above D6 level.
The *FALSE* answer is:
A. Leukocytosis is a reliable diagnostic clue.
B. Presence of urinary tract infection may delay the diagnosis.
C. Abdominal muscle rigidity is usually absent.
D. Tenderness is usually absent.
E. Autonomic dysreflexia is the most important sign.

✅ **Answer A**
- The laboratory findings including leukocytosis are not reliable. Many patients show leukocyturia at some stages with leukocytosis attributed mainly to UTI.

? 5. Vertebral artery injuries following cervical spine trauma.
The *FALSE* answer is:
A. High mortality rate if untreated.
B. Most common site is C1-C2.
C. Anticoagulation improves outcomes.
D. Digital subtraction angiography (DSA) detects BCVI in up to 34% of asymptomatic patients with blunt trauma.
E. In unstable fractures, early surgical fixation will prevent arterial damage.

✅ **Answer B**
- The point of entrance of the vertebral artery into the transverse foramen of C6 is the most common injured site followed by the C1-C2 site.

? 6. Autonomic dysfunction with spinal cord injuries above D6 level.
The *FALSE* answer is:
A. Neurogenic shock is due to impairment of parasympathetic influence.
B. Bradyarrhythmias are common in the acute phase.
C. Autonomic dysreflexia is common after 4–5 weeks post injury.
D. Full bladder may trigger autonomic dysreflexia.
E. Vagal hypersensitivity may occur in the acute phase.

✅ **Answer A**
- Neurogenic shock is due to impairment of sympathetic tone with intact parasympathetic influence by the vagal nerve.

❓ 7. Cervical spine injury associated with maxillofacial trauma.
The _FALSE_ answer is:
A. High-velocity maxillofacial facture is associated with higher incidence of cervical injury.
B. Spinal cord injury is more common in mixed (mandibular and non-mandibular) injuries.
C. Higher incidence in road traffic accidents.
D. Cord injury most common at the C1/C2 level.
E. Injuries to the lower cervical spine segments are associated with middle third facial fractures.

✔️ Answer D
▬ The C6/C7 level is most commonly injured, followed by C1/C2.

❓ 8. Facial fractures.
The _FALSE_ answer is:
A. Maxillary fracture is the most common indication for surgery.
B. Closed nasal fractures are the commonest.
C. The diagnosis of TON is primarily clinical.
D. Fractures extending to superior orbital fissure associated with ptosis.
E. Cribriform plate involvement associated cerebrospinal fluid leak.

✔️ Answer A
▬ Mandibular fracture is the commonest facial bone fracture that requires surgery.

❓ 9. Craniofacial trauma.
The _FALSE_ answer is:
A. Frontal sinus fractures imply severe trauma.
B. TBI is common in complex facial trauma.
C. CSF leak: the most common fracture site is the ethmoid sinus.
D. CSF leak: the second most common fracture site is the sphenoid sinus.
E. CSF leak responds well to conservative management.

✔️ Answer C
▬ The most common fracture site leak is the frontal sinus followed by sphenoid sinus with an incidence of 30.8% and 11.4–30.8%, respectively. The ethmoid sinus fracture site shows a lower incidence of leak of about 15.4–19.1%.

? 10. **Frontal sinus fractures.**
   The *FALSE* answer is:
   A. Posterior table is more resistant to injury than anterior table.
   B. Requires greater force to fracture than any other facial bone.
   C. Majority involve both anterior and posterior table.
   D. Indication for surgery in anterior table surgery is cosmesis.
   E. Sinus cranialization is used in displaced posterior wall fractures.

✓ **Answer A**
   − Anterior table is more resistant as it is much thicker.

? 11. **Intracranial complications of inadequately managed frontal sinus fractures.**
   The *FALSE* answer is:
   A. Mucocele.
   B. Rhinorrhea.
   C. Lateral sinus thrombosis.
   D. Brain abscess.
   E. Tension pneumocephalus.

✓ **Answer C**
   − Lateral sinus thrombosis (right or left transverse sinuses) is a complication of middle ear infection.

? 12. **Le Fort fractures.**
   The *FALSE* answer is:
   A. Le Fort I is more associated with CSF leak.
   B. Ruled out by absence of pterygoid fracture.
   C. Alcohol use associated with severe fracture types.
   D. Paranasal sinus effusions suggest fractures.
   E. Associated with hard palate fractures.

✓ **Answer A**
   − Le Fort II and III are most associated with CSF leak.

? **13. Facial gunshot injuries.**
   The *FALSE* answer is:
   A. 17% show altered mental status.
   B. 8% have concomitant spinal cord injury.
   C. Wounding capacity of a missile is directly related to its kinetic energy.
   D. Missile mass has greater impact on energy than velocity.
   E. Elastic tissues are more accommodating.

✓ Answer D
   ▬ Velocity has the greatest impact, as kinetic energy is calculated by the equation ($KE = \frac{1}{2}$ mass $\times$ velocity^2).

? **14. Sport-related TBI.**
   The *FALSE* answer is:
   A. Rarely fatal.
   B. 80% self-resolve within 10 days.
   C. Irritability points to concussion.
   D. Acute subdural hematoma usually associated with cerebral contusions.
   E. Persistent headache is an indication for cerebral imaging.

✓ Answer D
   ▬ The majority of ASDHs due to sport-related head injuries are simple ASDHs without cerebral contusion.

? **15. Sport-related SCI.**
   The *FALSE* answer is:
   A. Diving: most common cause.
   B. American football: cervical injury common.
   C. Complete paraplegia: most common neurological outcome at discharge.
   D. Rugby: most common level is C4–C6.
   E. Diving: most common level is C4.

✓ Answer C
   ▬ Incomplete tetraplegia is the most common neurological outcome at discharge, followed by complete tetraplegia, incomplete paraplegia, and complete paraplegia, respectively.

? 16. Brain death criteria.
   The *FALSE* answer is:
   A. Irreversible coma.
   B. Loss of corneal reflex.
   C. EEG is affected by drug intoxication.
   D. No somatosensory evoked potentials.
   E. Somatosensory evoked potentials less affected by hypothermia.

✓ Answer E
   ‒ Somatosensory evoked potentials less effected by drug intoxication but still affected by hypothermia.

? 17. Vegetative and minimally conscious patients: ethical issues.
   The *FALSE* answer is:
   A. Error rate in diagnosis is 43%.
   B. Functional MRI (fMRI) is used to detect residual cognitive function.
   C. Neuroimaging used to communicate with patients.
   D. Neuroimaging used in life-sustaining therapy decisions.
   E. Electroencephalography (EEG) has no role in detecting residual cognitive function.

✓ Answer E
   ‒ EEG, along with neuroimaging, is used detect residual cognitive function and even conscious awareness in both conditions.
   ‒ The ethical issues are related to the vulnerability of patients and families, difficulties to deal with negative results, restriction of communication to "yes" or "no" answers, and cost.

? 18. Awareness in the vegetative state.
   The *FALSE* answer is:
   A. Complete lack of cognitive function.
   B. Periods of wakefulness.
   C. EEG is superior to fMRI in detecting awareness.
   D. Movement artifacts are common in fMRI.
   E. EEG recordings are affected by metallic implants.

✓ Answer E
   ‒ EEG is superior to fMRI in detecting awareness as it is not affected by metallic implants.

? **19. Dead Donor Rule.**
The *FALSE* answer is:
A. Death declaration prior to donation.
B. Permanent cessation of all brain functions.
C. Permanent cessation of respiration and circulation.
D. Living donors always forbidden.
E. Is neither a law nor a regulation.

✓ Answer D
- Living donors are acceptable in pairing organs as donating one kidney under specific regulations (e.g., donating to a spouse).

? **20. TBI. Sleep disorders.**
The *FALSE* answer is:
A. Common.
B. More hours needed for sleep.
C. More prevalent in mild than moderate.
D. Result from diffuse axonal injury.
E. Direct and indirect brain injury.

✓ Answer C
- Sleep disorders are more frequent in moderate than mild TBI.
- Pathophysiology of post TBI involves different types of injuries, including but not limited to, diffuse axonal injury.

? **21. Major Depressive Disorder.**
The *FALSE* answer is:
A. High prevalence.
B. Associated with recurrent concussions.
C. High association with anxiety disorders.
D. Anti-cytokine treatment may reduce depression.
E. Selective serotonin receptor inhibitors (SSRIs) enhance cognition.

✓ Answer E
In the TBI population, randomized control trials (RCTs) on the efficacy of SSRIs have been few and limited to the specific outcome measures of depression and cognition. SSRI use is generally associated with improvements in depressive symptoms, although this effect may be a result of natural cerebral recovery. Conversely, SSRI administration was not found to have any benefit on cognition; in fact, it may worsen cognitive function

? 22. TBI. Hypertension.
   The *FALSE* answer is:
   A. Catecholamine excess is the main mechanism.
   B. Early exposure to beta-blockers reduces mortality.
   C. Catecholamine excess is associated with poor outcome.
   D. Catecholamine reduction is beneficial.
   E. Good outcomes in the pediatric age group.

✓ Answer E
   - Hypertension is frequent in pediatric age group, is often severe, and is strongly associated with increased mortality during the first 24 hours.

? 23. TBI. Catecholamine excess.
   The *FALSE* answer is:
   A. Regulates cerebral perfusion pressure.
   B. Initial catecholamine response is related to poor outcomes.
   C. Linked to neurogenic pulmonary edema.
   D. Triggered by elevation of intracranial pressure.
   E. Associated with cardiac dysfunction.

✓ Answer B
   - The initial catecholamine response may be protective through regulation of cerebral perfusion pressure.

? 24. TBI. Paroxysmal sympathetic hyperactivity.
   The *FALSE* answer is:
   A. Associated with severe TBI.
   B. Occurs in response to external stimuli.
   C. Associated with worse functional outcomes.
   D. High prevalence.
   E. More commonly associated with cortical and subcortical injuries than with deeper brain injuries.

✓ Answer E
   - Deeper brain injuries such as those affecting the periventricular white matter, corpus callosum, diencephalon, or brainstem are more likely to develop paroxysmal sympathetic hyperactivity than patients with cortical and subcortical injuries.

? 25. TBI. Cytokine changes.
The _FALSE_ answer is:
A. IL-6 peaks in the first 24 hours.
B. High levels linked to depression.
C. TGF-β increases.
D. TNF-α increases.
E. Elevation correlates with injury severity.

✓ Answer C
- TGF-β, a multifunctional cytokine, shows no significant dysregulation following TBI.

? 26. Orbital trauma.
The _FALSE_ answer is:
A. Subconjunctival hemorrhage is a common manifestation.
B. Greenstick orbital fractures associated with "trap-door" phenomenon.
C. Examination of the facial sensation is essential in all cases.
D. Le Forte fractures type I, II, and III are often associated with orbital trauma.
E. Associated with bradycardia in pediatrics.

✓ Answer D
- Not associated with Le Fort I.
- In children, orbital trauma may result in greenstick orbital fractures due to the elastic nature of bones. The fractured bone segment hinges on one side with the propensity of recoiling back. When the bone segment recoils back to its original position, it may impinge on the inferior rectus or orbital fat, and this is called the "trap-door" phenomenon. Constant pressure on the muscle may lead to oculocardiac reflex, manifesting with bradycardia, nausea, vomiting, and syncope.

? 27. Periorbital edema and ecchymosis.
The _FALSE_ answer is:
A. In children, consider shaken baby syndrome.
B. Usually indicate a serious injury.
C. Eyelids must be opened to evaluate for globe injury.
D. Ocular ultrasonography (B-scan) used to assess globe injury.
E. MRI of the orbit is sometimes indicated.

✅ **Answer B**
- Periorbital/periocular edema and ecchymosis are the most common presenting signs of blunt trauma to the eyelid, orbit, or forehead. They are generally innocuous signs, but careful evaluation is required to exclude serious associated injuries: globe injury, orbital fractures, and basal skull fracture.
- Ultrasonography may be useful in the detection of intraocular foreign bodies, globe rupture, suprachoroidal hemorrhage, and retinal detachment; it should be performed as gently as possible if there is the risk of an open globe injury, strictly avoiding any pressure on the globe.

❓ **28. Blow-out orbital fractures.**
  The *FALSE* answer is:
  A. Mostly caused by blunt trauma.
  B. Mostly involve the orbital floor.
  C. Subcutaneous emphysema associated with lateral wall fractures.
  D. The mechanism of diplopia is muscle entrapment.
  E. White-eyed fractures are seen in children.

✅ **Answer C**
- Subcutaneous emphysema occurs with fractures of medial wall and orbital floor which are in close relation with ethmoid and maxillary air sinuses, respectively. It typically develops on nose blowing, so in any case of orbital trauma with suspicion of orbital wall fracture, the patient is instructed not to blow his/her nose.
- White-eyed blow-out fracture is a condition that is seen in children who have orbital wall fracture but no periorbital soft tissue signs and no conjunctival congestion or hemorrhage.

❓ **29. Isolated orbital roof fractures.**
  The *FALSE* answer is:
  A. Rare type of orbital wall fractures.
  B. More common in adults.
  C. Caused by minor blunt trauma to the forehead.
  D. Associated with pneumocephalus.
  E. Treatment not always required.

✅ **Answer B**
- Isolated orbital roof fractures are more common in young children, in whom the frontal sinus has yet to pneumatize. Because the ratio of the cranial vault to the midface is greater in children than in adults. By contrast, frontal trauma in older individuals is partially absorbed by the frontal sinus, which diffuses the force and prevents extension of the fracture along the orbital roof.

❓ 30. Orbital floor fractures.
The *FALSE* answer is:
A. Enophthalmos is a late sign.
B. Orbital CT scan is the test of choice.
C. Diplopia is both upgaze and downgaze.
D. Fractures involving one-half of the orbital floor may be treated conservatively.
E. Patients with oculocardiac reflex must be operated on within 24–48 hours.

✅ Answer E
Patients with oculocardiac reflex must be operated on immediately to relieve the compression on the impinged muscle. Delayed treatment of oculocardiac reflex may lead to severe bradycardia, and even asystole.

❓ 31. Traumatic orbital hemorrhage.
The *FALSE* answer is:
A. Signs: afferent pupillary defect.
B. Signs: tight orbit.
C. Orbital compartment syndrome due to retrobulbar hemorrhage.
D. Orbital compartment syndrome: rapidly progressive vision loss.
E. Surgical decompression with lateral canthotomy is usually sufficient.

✅ Answer E
▬ Surgical decompression is most easily achieved by lateral canthotomy and cantholysis, in which the eyelids are disinserted from the lateral orbital rim, allowing the orbital volume to expand anteriorly. Lateral canthotomy alone does not sufficiently decrease orbital pressure; inferior cantholysis and sometimes superior cantholysis are also required.

❓ 32. Intraorbital foreign body.
The *FALSE* answer is:
A. Should be suspected in cases of penetrating trauma.
B. Orbital ultrasonography for objects positioned more anteriorly.
C. Organic foreign body: CT orbit.
D. Vegetable foreign bodies should be removed.
E. Foreign body in close proximity to the optic nerve can be left in place.

✅ **Answer C**

- Intraorbital foreign body can be organic (wood or vegetable matter) or inorganic (metallic, glass, or plastic matter). Wood and plastic foreign bodies are radiolucent on CT scan and radiopaque on MRI. However, MRI should be avoided if there is a possibility that the foreign object is ferromagnetic.
- Foreign bodies can be safely observed without surgery if they are inert and have smooth edges or if located in the posterior orbit or in close proximity to vital structures such as the optic nerve.
- Indications of intraorbital foreign body removal are as follows:
  1. Organic foreign bodies.
  2. Any foreign body regardless of its matter causing squint (due to interference with an extraocular muscle), inflammation, or infection.
  3. Anteriorly located foreign bodies.

❓ **33. Eyelid injuries.**
   The _FALSE_ answer is:
   A. Full-thickness injuries are classified as complicated.
   B. Orbit, globe, and optic nerve injuries are associations to be excluded.
   C. Eyelid wound repair should be done immediately.
   D. Orbital imaging is indicated in orbital wall fractures.
   E. Ptosis is a reported complication.

✅ **Answer C**

- Eyelid injuries may occur in the setting of multisystem trauma, the basic ABCs of the trauma management should be considered and ophthalmic evaluation and management deferred until more serious problems are addressed and the patient is stable.
- Globe injuries should be addressed first, and eyelid wound repair can be delayed up to 48 hours following trauma.
- The following eyelid injuries are considered complicated: full-thickness, has a ruptured globe, presence of intraorbital foreign body, involving the lacrimal draining system, involving the levator aponeurosis or superior rectus muscle, has a damage to the lid margin, has a visible orbital fat prolapse, includes medial canthal tendon rupture, or extensive tissue loss.

❷ 34. Eyelid lacerations.
The *FALSE* answer is:
A. Partial-thickness lacerations involve the skin and orbicularis muscle.
B. Full-thickness lacerations usually involve the lid margin.
C. Canalicular injury is suspected when a lower lid laceration lies medial to the inferior punctum.
D. In upper lid laceration, orbital fat prolapse indicates orbital septum injury.
E. Orbital septum lacerations should always be repaired.

✅ Answer E
- Care should be taken not to incorporate or suture the opened orbital septum to avoid upper eyelid retraction and tethering to the superior orbital rim by vertical shortening of the sutured orbital septum. When the orbital septum is injured, it is important to explore the levator muscle and aponeurosis and repair any laceration to prevent ptosis.

❷ 35. Surgical reconstruction of traumatic eyelid defects.
The *FALSE* answer is:
A. Small (<5 mm) full thickness defects: healing by secondary intention.
B. Small defects of less than one third of the horizontal eyelid length: direct closure.
C. Defect is too large for direct closure and is less than one third of the horizontal eyelid length: lateral canthotomy and cantholysis.
D. Medium defects of up to half of the horizontal eyelid length: flap.
E. Large defects of more than half of the horizontal length of the lid: graft.

✅ Answer A
- Healing by secondary intention or granulation (laissez-faire) is considered for small (<5 mm) partial thickness defects or defects near the canthi.

❷ 36. Indications of orbital CT scan in eyelid and orbital trauma.
The *FALSE* answer is:
A. Suspicion of intraorbital foreign body.
B. Crepitus on palpation of the orbital rim.
C. Step deformity in the upper eyelid.
D. Inability to elevate the eye with diplopia.
E. Subconjunctival hemorrhage.

✅ **Answer E**
- Usually, a subconjunctival hemorrhage is not an indication for CT scan unless it is diffuse without a visible posterior limit, which may indicate an orbital wall fracture in a patient sustained a severe trauma.
- On palpation of the orbital rim, a step indicates displaced orbital rim fracture, while crepitus or crackling sensation indicates subcutaneous emphysema occurs due to air in the subcutaneous tissues escaping from the adjacent paranasal air sinuses. These are signs of orbital wall fracture.
- Paresthesia in the lower eyelid, side of the nose, cheek, and upper lip and upper teeth is another indication.

❓ **37. Globe injuries.**
   The *FALSE* **answer is:**
   A. Closed globe injury is caused by blunt trauma.
   B. Globe rupture is open globe injury caused by blunt trauma.
   C. Penetrating injury refers to a single full-thickness wound.
   D. Perforation consists of two full-thickness wounds.
   E. Perforating injury is usually associated with intraocular foreign body.

✅ **Answer E**
Perforating injuries differ from penetrating injuries in that they have both entry and exit wounds in the former, while the latter has only entry wound. Penetrating injuries are usually associated with an intraocular foreign body.

❓ **38. Management of open globe injuries.**
   The *FALSE* **answer is:**
   A. Small corneal wounds can be treated conservatively.
   B. Intravenous antibiotics and pain killers are indicated.
   C. Intravitreal antibiotic injection is indicated.
   D. Surgical repair can be delayed up to 72 hours.
   E. General anesthesia is preferred.

✅ **Answer D**
- Surgery should occur as soon as possible to minimize further damage to the intraocular contents and prevent microbial proliferation and traumatic endophthalmitis (intraocular infection).
- Injuries associated with soil contamination and/or retained intraocular foreign bodies increase the risk of Bacillus endophthalmitis. Because this organism can destroy the eye within 24 hours, intravenous and/or intravitreal antibiotics (injection of antibiotics inside the vitreous cavity) should be considered.

? **39. Surgical repair of open globe injuries.**
The _FALSE_ answer is:
A. The primary goal is to preserve vision.
B. Repair of a corneoscleral laceration should take precedence over non-life-threatening surgical problems elsewhere on the body.
C. Repair of eyelid injuries should follow repair of the globe itself.
D. Unless frankly necrotic and macerated, a prolapsed intraocular tissue such as iris should be reposted back into the globe.
E. Primary enucleation is indicated is severely devastating injured globe.

✓ Answer A

■ The primary goal of the repair is to restore the integrity of the globe. The secondary goal at the time of the primary repair or during subsequent procedures is to restore vision.

■ Repair of eyelid injury should follow repair of the globe itself because eyelid surgery can put pressure on an open globe, and certain eyelid lacerations may actually improve globe exposure.

8

Suggested Reading

Al-Ameri LT, Mohsin TS, Abdul Wahid AT. Sleep disorders following mild and moderate traumatic brain injury. Brain Sci. 2019;9(1):10.

Al-Mujaini A, Al-Senawi R, Ganesh A, Al-Zuhaibi S, Al-Dhuhli H. Intraorbital foreign body: clinical presentation, radiological appearance and management. Sultan Qaboos Univ Med J. 2008;8(1):69.

Al-Thowaibi A, Kumar M, Al-Matani I. An overview of penetrating ocular trauma with retained intraocular foreign body. Saudi J Ophthalmol. 2011;25(2):203–5.

Ariyoshi Y, Naito H, Yumoto T, Iida A, Yamamoto H, Fujisaki N, Aokage T, Tsukahara K, Yamada T, Mandai Y, Osako T. Orbital emphysema as a consequence of forceful nose-blowing: report of a case. Case Rep Emerg Med. 2019;2019:4383086.

Aylward GW. Vitreous management in penetrating trauma: primary repair and secondary intervention. Eye. 2008;22(10):1366–9.

Bar-On Z, Ohry A. The acute abdomen in spinal cord injury individuals. Spinal Cord. 1995;33(12):704–6.

Blumenthal I. Shaken baby syndrome. Postgrad Med J. 2002;78(926):732–5.

Bodnar CN, Morganti JM, Bachstetter AD. Depression following a traumatic brain injury: uncovering cytokine dysregulation as a pathogenic mechanism. Neural Regen Res. 2018;13(10):1693.

Chan CW, Eng JJ, Tator CH, Krassioukov A, Spinal Cord Injury Research Evidence Team. Epidemiology of sport-related spinal cord injuries: a systematic review. J Spinal Cord Med. 2016;39(3):255–64.

Cochran ML, Czyz CN. Eyelid Laceration. StatPearls [Internet]. 2020.

Colby K. Management of open globe injuries. Int Ophthalmol Clin. 1999;39(1):59–69.

Cruse D, Chennu S, Chatelle C, Bekinschtein TA, Fernández-Espejo D, Pickard JD, Laureys S, Owen AM. Bedside detection of awareness in the vegetative state: a cohort study. Lancet. 2011;378(9809):2088–94.

Donald PJ. Neurosurgery: skull base craniofacial trauma. J Neurolog Surg B Skull Base. 2016;77(5):412.

Gupta S, Kumar A. Child abuse: inflicted traumatic brain injury. Indian Pediatr. 2007;44(10):783.

Hada M. Eyelid reconstruction techniques: an overview. Off Sci J Delhi Ophthalmol Soc. 2018;28(3):51–4.

Hagen EM. Acute complications of spinal cord injuries. World J Orthop. 2015;6(1):17.

Johnson MA, Borgman MA, Cannon JW, Kuppermann N, Neff LP. Severely elevated blood pressure and early mortality in children with traumatic brain injuries: the neglected end of the spectrum. West J Emerg Med. 2018;19(3):452.

Karki KT, Nepal PR. Predictors and significance of orbital fracture in traumatic brain injury. Eastern Green Neurosurg. 2020;2(1):18–22.

Kaufman Y, Cole P, Hollier LH. Facial gunshot wounds: trends in management. Craniomaxillofac Trauma Reconstr. 2009;2(2):85–90.

Krishnamoorthy V, Chaikittisilpa N, Kiatchai T, Vavilala M. Hypertension after severe traumatic brain injury: friend or foe? J Neurosurg Anesthesiol. 2017;29(4):382.

Lin KY, Ngai P, Echegoyen JC, Tao JP. Imaging in orbital trauma. Saudi J Ophthalmol. 2012;26(4):427–32.

Manara AR. All human death is brain death: the legacy of the Harvard criteria. Resuscitation. 2019;138:210–2.

Metzinger SE, Metzinger RC. Complications of frontal sinus fractures. Craniomaxillofac Trauma Reconstr. 2009;2(1):27–34.

Mizobuchi Y, Nagahiro S. A review of sport-related head injuries. Korean J Neurotrauma. 2016;12(1):1.

Mueller CA, Peters I, Podlogar M, Kovacs A, Urbach H, Schaller K, Schramm J, Kral T. Vertebral artery injuries following cervical spine trauma: a prospective observational study. Eur Spine J. 2011;20(12):2202–9.

Mukherjee S, Abhinav K, Revington PJ. A review of cervical spine injury associated with maxillofacial trauma at a UK tertiary referral centre. Ann R Coll Surg Engl. 2015;97(1): 66–72.

Oh JW, Kim SH, Whang K. Traumatic cerebrospinal fluid leak: diagnosis and management. Korean J Neurotrauma. 2017;13(2):63.

Pfeifer R, Teuben M, Andruszkow H, Barkatali BM, Pape HC. Mortality patterns in patients with multiple trauma: a systematic review of autopsy studies. PLoS One. 2016;11(2):e0148844.

Pham CM, Couch SM. Oculocardiac reflex elicited by orbital floor fracture and inferior globe displacement. Am J Ophthalmol Case Rep. 2017 Jun 1;6:4–6.

Phillips BJ, Turco LM. Le Fort fractures: a collective review. Bull Emerg Trauma. 2017; 5(4):221.

Roselló EG, Granado AM, Garcia MA, Martí SJ, Sala GL, Mármol BB, Gutiérrez SP. Facial fractures: classification and highlights for a useful report. Insights Imaging. 2020;11(1): 1–5.

Roth FS, Koshy JC, Goldberg JS, Soparkar CN. Pearls of orbital trauma management. Semin Plast Surg. Thieme Medical Publishers. 2010;24(4):398.

Sadashivam S. Isolated orbital roof fracture: can it be catastrophic? Asian J Neurosurg. 2018;13(3):935.

Sade RM. Brain death, cardiac death, and the dead donor rule. J S C Med Assoc (1975). 2011;107(4):146.

Turgut B, Karanfil FC, Turgut FA. Orbital compartment syndrome. Beyoglu Eye J. 2019;4(1):1–4.

Vezzani A, Viviani B. Neuromodulatory properties of inflammatory cytokines and their impact on neuronal excitability. Neuropharmacology. 2015;96:70–82.

Weijer C, Peterson A, Webster F, Graham M, Cruse D, Fernández-Espejo D, Gofton T, Gonzalez-Lara LE, Lazosky A, Naci L, Norton L. Ethics of neuroimaging after serious brain injury. BMC Med Ethics. 2014;15(1):1–3.

Weiner M, Bedrossiam EH. Eyelid trauma. Della Rocca RC, Bedrossiam EH, Arthurs BP, editors. New York: McGraw Hill. 2002. p. 157–161.

Zheng RZ, Lei ZQ, Yang RZ, Huang GH, Zhang GM. Identification and management of paroxysmal sympathetic hyperactivity after traumatic brain injury. Front Neurol. 2020;11:81.

8

Supplementary Information

Suggested Reading Book List – 168

Suggested Reading Book List

▬ The General Neurosurgery Textbooks
- Youmans J, Winn H. Youmans & Winn neurological surgery. 7th ed. Philadelphia: Elsevier; 2017.
- Greenberg M. Handbook of neurosurgery. 9th ed. New York, USA: Thieme Medical Publishers; 2019.
- Shaffrey C, Couldwell W, Harbaugh R. Neurosurgery knowledge update: a comprehensive review. Thieme Medical Publishers Incorporated; 2015.
- Steinmetz M, Benzel E. Benzel's spine surgery. Philadelphia: Elsevier; 2017.
- Thamburaj V. Textbook of contemporary neurosurgery. Vols 1 & 2. New Delhi: Japee Brothers Medical Publishers; 2013.

▬ Cranial Neurotrauma
- Tsao J. Traumatic brain injury. 2nd ed. New York, USA: Springer; 2019.
- Jallo J, Loftus C. Neurotrauma and critical care of the brain. 2nd ed. New York, USA: Thieme Medical Publishers; 2018.
- Abelson-Mitchell N. Neurotrauma: Managing patients with head injury. 1st ed. John Wiley & Sons; 2013.
- Kobeissy F. Brain neurotrauma. Boca Raton: CRC Press; 2015.
- Whitfield P, Thomas E, Summers F, Whyte M, Hutchinson P. Head injury. Cambridge: Cambridge University Press; 2009.
- Mahapatra A, Kamal R. Textbook of head injury. 4th ed. New Delhi, India: CBS Pub- lishers and Distributors Pvt Ltd; 2014.

▬ Spinal Neurotrauma
- Jallo J, Vaccaro A. Neurotrauma and critical care of the spine. 2nd ed. New York, USA: Thieme Medical Publishers; 2018.

▬ Others
- Lo E, Lok J, Ning M, Whalen M. Vascular mechanisms in CNS trauma. New York, USA: Springer; 2014.

- Di Saverio S, Balogh Z. Trauma management, trauma critical care, orthopaedic trauma and neuro-trauma. Springer; 2014.
- Jallo J, Urtecho J. The Jefferson manual for neurocritical care. 1st ed. New York, USA: Thieme Medical Publishers; 2021.
- Pryll J, Raksin P, Ullman J. Atlas of emergency neurosurgery. New York: Thieme Medical Publishers; 2015.
- Weber J, Maas A. Neurotrauma. 1st ed. New York, USA: Elsevier; 2007.
- Madden C. Neurotrauma (Neurosurgery by example book 8). 1st ed. New York, USA: Oxford University Press; 2020.
- Ecklund J, Moores L. Neurotrauma management for the severely injured polytrauma patient. 1st ed. Cham, Germany: Springer; 2017.
- Valadka A, Andrews B. Neurotrauma. New York: Thieme Medical Publishers; 2005.
- Handbook on the neuropsychology of traumatic brain injury. 1st ed. [Place of publication not identified]: Springer; 2015.
- Silver J. Textbook of traumatic brain injury. 3rd ed. Washington, USA: American Psychiatric Publishing, Inc.; 2018.